Trans Women and HIV

"In the face of high levels of stigmatisation and prejudice against trans people, this book offers an important contribution to knowledge. It takes a nuanced and insightful approach to a neglected area—trans women and HIV—and it will be of interest to practitioners, policy makers, and those who are concerned with health, sexuality, and gender."

—Prof. Surya Monro, *University of Huddersfield, UK*

"As a psychological practitioner providing clinical education and training to the next generation of mental health workers, I believe that this timely and relevant book highlights the importance of understanding the phenomenological perspective of sexual and ethnic diversity in the medical and psychiatric models. The case studies bring to life the people behind the labels, integrating the context and theoretical foundations to provide an empathic, resilience-based model to promote psycho-medical well-being interventions. This book also offers a way forward with recommendations for policy makers and programme developers managing health risks and health promotion."

—Dr. Joann Griffith, *De Montfort University, Leicester, UK*

"Trans women living with HIV may be uncounted in datasets. This book details exquisitely the complex intersectional aspects of stigma faced by this group, exposing its structurally violent and disempowering nature. Jaspal notes the struggle to construct an identity characterised by "self-esteem, continuity, belonging and authenticity", compounded by HIV status, and the coping mechanisms that may be adopted to deal with transphobia, sexism and racism. It is a powerful and essential work, and for clinicians offers important, practical recommendations that we must strive better to embed into HIV care and prevention services. We are left with a key question needing urgent attention—how can we all discourage concealment and self-isolation among trans women living with HIV, to reduce stigma, and improve health overall?"

—Dr. Tristan J. Barber, *Royal Free Hospital, London, UK*

Rusi Jaspal

Trans Women and HIV

Social Psychological Perspectives

palgrave
macmillan

Rusi Jaspal
School of Social Sciences
Nottingham Trent University
Nottingham, UK

ISBN 978-3-030-57544-1   ISBN 978-3-030-57545-8   (eBook)
https://doi.org/10.1007/978-3-030-57545-8

This Palgrave Macmillan imprint is published by the registered company Springer Nature Switzerland AG
The registered company address is: Gewerbestrasse 11, 6330 Cham, Switzerland

ACKNOWLEDGEMENTS

My research career has seen me explore aspects of identity, relationships and psychological wellbeing in many minority groups in society. Throughout all of these research projects, I have always been motivated by the same things: my deep appreciation of diversity, which enriches our society; my fascination with the functioning of social groups; and my conviction that diversity must be supported so that minority groups can thrive and flourish. Outgroups have a crucial role to play in enabling minority groups to experience social and psychological wellbeing. It has felt very rewarding to write this book about transgender women living with HIV in the UK. The book begins to fill a gap that many of us in the field of HIV have long lamented. I am immensely grateful to the eleven trans women who generously shared their experiences with me. I thank my Ph.D. students over the years whose ideas have inspired me. I would like to express my deepest gratitude to Aedan J Wolton without whose support this project would simply not have come to fruition. I am grateful to Lauren Kennedy who was my research assistant on the EXTRA (Experiences of Trans Women Living With HIV) Study and to Sue Hayward who provided excellent administrative support. I thank my beloved family—Ramesh, Asha, Babak and Jaya—for their unwavering support during the writing of this and other books.

CONTENTS

LIST OF FIGURES

PART I

Trans Women in Context

CHAPTER 1

Understanding Trans Women and HIV

Abstract In this introductory chapter, the social psychological focus of the volume on the experiences, identities and psychological well-being of trans women living with HIV in the UK is discussed. The key questions addressed in this volume are described: (1) How do trans women living with HIV experience their diagnosis and the 'stressors' associated with the condition? (2) How do they perceive and manage HIV disclosure? (3) How does the experience of living with HIV shape identity and psychological well-being among trans women? Two case studies are provided to illustrate the psychological challenges among trans women living with HIV in the UK. Key terms that are used in the volume are defined. A brief history of trans women and a brief overview of key statistics on the trans population and of HIV incidence in the UK are provided.

Keywords HIV · Trans women · Trans history · HIV epidemiology · Social psychology

The field of human immunodeficiency virus (HIV) has undergone significant development since the first clinical observations of acquired immune deficiency syndrome (AIDS) in 1981. HIV has gone from being an almost invariably life-limiting disease to a life-changing chronic condition. Effective treatments have been developed, ensuring a very good prognosis for those diagnosed and treated early. Both the efficacy and tolerability of

© The Author(s) 2020
R. Jaspal, *Trans Women and HIV*,
https://doi.org/10.1007/978-3-030-57545-8_1

treatments have improved considerably over the years. HIV testing is widespread. More recently, unequivocal evidence has emerged showing that patients on effective antiretroviral therapy (ART) who have an undetectable HIV viral load cannot infect their sexual partners—popularly referred to as 'undetectable=untransmittable' or 'U=U'. With the advent of pre-exposure prophylaxis (PrEP), an additional highly effective layer of protection against the virus has emerged.

These impressive developments in HIV medicine have paved the way for the ambitious aspiration, and genuine belief, that HIV can be eliminated. In 2014, the Joint United Nations Programme on HIV/AIDS (UNAIDS) set the ambitious 90-90-90 target, that is, for 90% of people living with HIV to be aware of their positive serostatus, for 90% of them to be on effective treatment, and for 90% of patients with diagnosed HIV to have an undetectable viral load. In 2018, it was confirmed that the United Kingdom (UK) had surpassed these targets, achieving 92-98-97, respectively (Public Health England, 2019). In 2019, Matt Hancock, the UK Secretary of State for Health and Social Care, declared the UK's commitment to end all new HIV transmissions by 2030.[1] Collectively, medical innovation, institutional commitment, and public aspiration may well make this commitment a reality. Yet, there remain at least two significant challenges to achieving this ambitious target, which constitute the foci of this volume.

First, it is clear that, while HIV patients are increasingly enjoying better physical health outcomes as a result of developments in HIV medicine, the unabating insidious stigma that surrounds the virus continues to cause psychological distress to those diagnosed and living with HIV. What is the impact of an HIV diagnosis on the identity of the individual? How does it affect their psychological well-being? How do HIV patients in distress cope and, perhaps more importantly, how can they be supported to cope effectively? These questions are important because existing research suggests that people with decreased psychological well-being are at greater risk of poor health outcomes (Jaspal & Lopes, 2020).

Second, not all groups in society experience HIV in quite the same way. There is evidence of health inequalities in minority groups—along

---

[1] https://www.gov.uk/government/news/health-secretary-announces-goal-to-end-hiv-transmissions-by-2030.

the usual fault lines of ethnicity, sexuality and gender. Trans women—a key population in the HIV epidemic—face a major burden in relation to HIV infection. Global data show that they are much more likely to acquire HIV and that those who do are much less likely to be diagnosed early, to receive and adhere to treatment, and to experience as good a prognosis as patients from other groups in society (see Chapter 3). Trans women experience many other social and psychological stressors which can put them at disproportionately high risk of HIV but also of poorer general health outcomes.

This book focuses on the experiences, identities and psychological wellbeing of trans women living with HIV in the UK. It explores theory and research into HIV among trans women, on the one hand, and examines interview data from a sample of trans women living with HIV in the UK, on the other hand. Three key questions lie at the heart of this volume:

- How do trans women living with HIV experience their diagnosis and the 'stressors' associated with the condition?
- How do they perceive and manage HIV disclosure?
- How does the experience of living with HIV shape identity and psychological wellbeing among trans women?

Case Studies

In order to illustrate the significance of these questions, two case studies of trans women living with HIV are presented. The cases are real but individuals' names have been replaced by pseudonyms and some details have been changed to prevent identification:

Case Study 1: Sally, a 51-Year-Old Trans Woman Living with HIV

Sally was assigned male sex at birth but, even as a child, felt like a girl. She never attempted to explain these feelings to her family or friends because she did not know how to and thought they wouldn't understand. As an adolescent, Sally felt attracted to boys and thought that she might be gay. At the time, this was not socially acceptable but it felt more acceptable than telling people that she felt like a girl. Sally was rejected by her parents and bullied by her peers. She felt very lonely. At the age of 18, Sally left home and decided to transition away from her family. She met her former partner Jim with whom she started to use alcohol and recreational drugs. She became involved in sex work so that they could maintain their lifestyle. During the course of her work, Sally was violently assaulted several times. In the early 90s, Jim died of AIDS and that year Sally also tested positive for HIV. This added a further layer of complexity to her already complex life. Given that no HIV treatments were available at the time, Sally was told that she would probably not survive for much longer. Desolate and bereft, she confided in a friend who was sympathetic but concerned about catching HIV through even casual contact with her. Sally managed to survive long enough to receive HIV treatment when it was introduced in 1996. Although Sally is in relatively good physical health, she still feels traumatised by her near-death experience. She feels lonely and isolated and, given that she has never really been supported by others, is mistrustful of others. This is further compounded by the fact that she is often ridiculed by people in the street because she does not pass as a cisgender woman.

Case Study 2: Pritika, a 25-Year-Old Trans Woman Living with HIV

Pritika was born in India and moved to London to study at university. Pritika concealed from her parents the fact that she was trans because of the stigma surrounding hijras[2] in India. When she started her university education, Pritika joined the lesbian, gay, bisexual and trans (LGBT) student society and befriended Jess, a trans woman, in whom she confided. Jess shared with Pritika her own story of transitioning at the age of 18 and provided her with support to begin her own gender transition. Away from her parents in India, Pritika felt empowered to think seriously about transitioning. Pritika went to see her GP but soon became frustrated with her GP's response and the time the process was taking. Healthcare professionals did not seem to believe what she was telling them and kept on asking her if she was sure about her feelings. Dismayed at the medical response, she purchased hormones online and began to self-medicate. After a few months, she noticed some significant bodily changes which made her appearance feel more aligned to her gender identity. Pritika also met her boyfriend on a mobile social networking application and they developed a sexual relationship, rarely using condoms. She was not particularly knowledgeable about the

---

[2] Hijras are legally recognised as a third gender in various South Asian countries (Agrawal, 1997). Some are intersex but most were assigned male sex at birth but identify as hijra. Hijras can be regarded as trans.

risk of HIV given that the topic was never really discussed in India. A few months later, Pritika tested positive for HIV during a routine sexual health screening organised at her university. Her test result was confirmed at the local sexual health clinic and she was encouraged to begin HIV medication. However, Pritika was nervous about beginning treatment because of what she had heard about side effects and, especially, what the implications might be for her gender transition. Pritika preferred to focus on her transition, felt that her doctor was not understanding towards her and thus decided not to return to the clinic. She also broke up with her boyfriend and felt unable to tell him that she had HIV because she thought that he might blame her. Pritika feels that she has nobody to speak to.

These case studies are not intended to be representative of trans women's experiences of living with HIV. Rather, they are supposed to be illustrative of some of the challenges that may be faced by trans women who are diagnosed with the condition. The case studies evoke issues of identity, family relationships, social support, bullying, homophobia, transphobia, violence, sex work, medical mistrust, perceived risk of drug interactions, risk and several others. Many of these issues are discussed more extensively in the rest of this volume. The case studies exhibit the complex lives of trans women living with HIV who may be grappling not only with the social psychological stressors associated with their gender identity but also with those prompted by their HIV status.

The case studies are intended to show that some trans women are living with HIV in precarious social and psychological circumstances, devoid of essential social and clinical support. The reasons for decreased support are multifarious—some trans women are rejected and victimised due to their identity, while others pre-emptively opt for isolation in order to protect themselves from stigma. Social and cultural context is key to predicting how individuals will cope with adversity, such as an HIV diagnosis. While Sally grew up during an era in which acknowledging her trans identity was difficult, the culture in which Pritika was socialised was prohibitively transphobic. In this volume, the experiences of trans women living with HIV are explored through a social psychological lens. This is intended to elucidate how social context and individual experience interact to produce particular psychological and physical health outcomes for individuals in this population.

DEFINITIONS

It is important to define what is meant by the key terms used in this volume. Accordingly, the gender identity terms (such as trans and cisgender), the notion of gender transitioning, identity, and psychological wellbeing are defined. These terms are used differently in the literature and, thus, require some commentary in the interest of clarity.

Gender Identity Terms

Many different terms are used to describe gender identity. In this volume, the term 'trans' is used as an inclusive term which encompasses a series of other more specific identities, such as 'transgender', 'transsexual', and 'cross dresser'. It is used to refer to the social and psychological state of non-alignment between the sex which one was assigned at birth and the gender with which one identifies. Nicolazzo (2016) has conceptualised the category trans as 'an open question pointing toward the instability of the assumed gender binary, recognizing trans* people as comprising a community of difference' (p. 16) and, thus, acknowledges the wide range of gender identities that this broad category encompasses.

People who identify as trans undergo a gender 'transition' of some sort. This may be physical in that a trans person may undergo hormone replacement therapy in order to develop physical characteristics consistent with the gender with which they identify. They may undergo gender reassignment surgery (orchidectomy) and have a vaginoplasty (in the case of female-to-male trans people). However, not all trans women decide to undergo gender reassignment surgery—as indicated in this study, some are happy to retain their masculine genitals while undergoing hormone replacement therapy. Some of the trans women who participated in this study had not undertaken a physical gender transition at all but had transitioned *psychologically* in that they self-identified as trans women. Furthermore, many had transitioned *socially* in that they also presented as female in some or all social contexts. Some trans women who transition psychologically and/or socially have not undergone any physical intervention as part of their gender transition. Some have no intention or desire to do so. In this volume, the generic term 'trans' is used as an umbrella category to capture all of these experiences, labels and identities.

The term 'cisgender' is used to refer to people whose gender identity is aligned with the sex assigned at birth. It is frequented used by trans people to refer to people who are 'not trans' (Pearce, 2018). It is noteworthy that some trans people also define themselves as 'non-binary', which acknowledges that it is not always possible to align one's identity to the binary categories of male and female (Matsuno & Budge, 2017). Non-binary individuals identify as neither male nor female and, thus, use a gender identity term which captures elements of both masculine and feminine experience. This gender identity term has become increasingly prevalent, with some individuals initially identifying binarily as trans women or men but later adopting a non-binary identity. However, the individuals who participated in this study identified (binarily) as trans women and, consequently, the experiences of non-binary trans people are not discussed or reported in this volume.

Gender Transitioning

There are many views on what 'transitioning' actually means. As demonstrated below, the Gender Recognition Act 2004 stipulates that seven key criteria must be met in order for a Gender Recognition Certificate to be issued. These relatively strict criteria are perhaps the reason why only 4910 people in the UK have had their gender identity officially recognised, despite the prediction that there are in fact hundreds of thousands of trans people in the UK (LGBT Policy Team, 2018). Some individuals have elected to have gender reassignment surgery—to varying degrees—in order to transition, while others take the decision solely to initiate hormone replacement theory. Some may do neither but 'present' as the gender with which they identify—again to varying degrees.

Consistent with the social psychological perspective taken in this volume, gender transitioning is understood as a social psychological process, that is, as a state of gender dysphoria which is accompanied by cognition, affect and behaviour to live in accordance with the gender with which one identifies. How one 'lives in accordance' with this gender is a fundamentally social psychological question. There are many social, psychological, economic, institutional and other factors that determine the measures taken in order to transition. They may have little, nothing or everything to do with gender identity. For Pritika in case study above, transitioning (in any visible manner) in India while living under the watchful eyes of her parents was perceived to be impossible. For Sally, gender reassignment surgery soon after her HIV diagnosis in the pre-ART era was deemed to be medically risky. Yet, they are both trans women and can both be said to have transitioned. We live in a world that consists of social norms, which determine who is perceived to have and not to have transitioned. It is important to view this social psychological issue from the perspective of the individual himself/herself and not through the lens of these social norms.

Identity

Identity can be defined in many ways depending on one's disciplinary approach. It can be thought of as an individual construct, that is, the individual's perception of who they are—a product of individual cognition and affect. It can also be conceptualised as a group membership, that is, self-definition primarily as a member of a particular social group. Furthermore, some scholars view identity as relatively stable, while others conceptualise it as being in constant flux.

How we define identity also depends on our epistemological approach (Jaspal & Breakwell, 2014). Social constructionists refer to identity as being 'constructed' in discourse while realists tend to describe it as an 'object' that can be perceived, described and observed using the right methods. There is merit in all of these approaches and they are not necessarily incompatible. It would perhaps be a theoretical limitation to focus on any specific approach to the detriment of others. Thus, in accordance with the social psychological perspective taken in this volume, identity is defined as the constellation of characteristics (personality traits, group memberships, emotions, behaviours) which comprise one's self-perception, which are derived from one's personal experience and relationships with other people (Breakwell, 1986).

Identity is influenced by the social context but manifested in thought and action. Society makes available the 'resources' for identity construction but the process of constructing identity is an interaction between cognition, affect and society. As we enter and leave social groups and as the social context evolves, our identity changes. Using the right analytic approaches, we can describe, understand and predict identity processes in any population. Consistent with identity process theory (see Chapter 2), an analysis of how trans women living with HIV respond to potential 'threats' to identity can shed light on the processes of identity construction in this population.

Psychological Wellbeing

The concept of *psychological wellbeing* is used to refer to a multitude of distinct but inter-related phenomena. In this volume, it is defined as the state of psychological equilibrium between the psychological stressors that one faces, on the one hand, and the social psychological resources that one possesses for dealing with these stressors, on the other hand (Jaspal, 2018). As outlined in the rest of this volume, people regularly face challenges (also thought of in terms of threats to identity), some of which are relatively trivial and transient and others which are more serious and chronic. In the context of HIV-positive trans women's lives, stressors may include misgendering, prejudice, an HIV diagnosis, and others. They are described as stressors because they can cause psychological stress and, thus, undermine one's state of psychological wellbeing. This may be described in terms of 'feeling down' or 'sad' or 'anxious' and so on. However, as indicated in Chapter 2, individuals cope with these stressors in a variety of ways—some adaptive and others maladaptive. There are many factors—both social and psychological—which determine the type of coping strategy that is available to the individual and employed by them. These factors can either extend or limit the individual's capacity to cope with the stressors. The ability to select strategies for coping effectively with challenges will in turn determine the extent to which the individual experiences psychological wellbeing. Conversely, the inability to cope effectively, due, for instance, to the absence of social support, will shift the equilibrium in favour of the stressor, thereby undermining psychological wellbeing. In short, psychological wellbeing is this 'balance' between psychological stress and coping.

THE ROLE OF SOCIAL PSYCHOLOGY

This book provides an analysis of the experiences of trans women living with HIV through a social psychological lens. Social psychology is best described as the meeting-point between psychology and sociology. If one thinks of psychology specifically as the examination of cognition, affect and behaviour in the individual and of sociology as the study of inter-personal relationships, society and institutions, social psychology can be located at the intersection of these two approaches (Jaspal & Breakwell, 2014).

More specifically, social psychology refers to the study of how individual cognition, affect and behaviour are shaped by one's (imagined or actual) interpersonal relationships, society and institutions. There is a long-standing tradition of social psychological research into the formation of attitudes; the construction of identity, that is, how one views oneself in relation to others; and the formation, operation and interaction of social groups. As demonstrated in the case studies above and in the chapters that follow, these issues are pertinent to the experiences of trans women living with HIV. Trans women living with HIV are struggling to construct an identity against a backdrop of culture, society and legal and healthcare institutions. Their self-image is shaped at least in part by the perceptions of others. Their attitudes towards HIV are affected by social stigma. The coping strategies that they develop are rooted in both psychological and social processes.

Social psychologists have examined these issues in a broad range of empirical settings and populations, which has led to the development of theories that may be generalised across populations. In Part I of this volume, tenets of theories from social psychology are outlined in relation to the experiences of trans women living with HIV and, in Part II, they are applied to the accounts of individuals living in the UK. In particular, identity process theory from social psychology lies at the heart of this volume and its tenets are used flexibly to add theoretical depth to the analysis of trans women's experiences of living, and coping, with HIV. The theory lays the foundations for the theoretical model for understanding and predicting responses to HIV in this population, which is outlined in Chapter 3.

A Brief History of Trans Women in the UK

The focus of this volume is on the experiences of trans women living with HIV in the UK. In order to understand these experiences, it is important to summarise briefly the history of trans women in the UK and, in particular, the social, psychological and legal aspects of this history. Several insightful texts have recently been published on this topic and should be consulted for a more thorough overview (e.g. Burns, 2018; Stryker, 2017). Although trans identity is often presented and understood as 'new', trans people have in fact existed for a long time. Due to stigma, decreased visibility, a lack of legal recognition, and slow medical advances in the field of gender identity, trans people have remained invisible in much of history and on the margins of society. This lack of visibility has further reinforced the stigma appended to transness.

There is a long-standing history of transvestism, that is, dressing in a manner that is socially represented as being more consistent with the opposite gender (to that assigned at birth). Transvestism is not synonymous with transgenderism although, in some cases, it could be seen as part of the 'trans umbrella'. People may transiently present as the opposite gender for a number of reasons that are unrelated to their gender identity—indeed, in some cultures, transvestism may be practised for cultural, religious or ceremonial purposes (Burns, 2018). It is also difficult to know how many transvestites in the past self-identified as trans, that is, whether they disidentified from the gender that they were assigned at birth and, thus, attempted to present in a manner that was consistent with their psychological gender. Similarly, in order to avoid social stigma and to gain social acceptance, some trans people (i.e. those who identified with a gender that is different from the sex assigned to them at birth) may never have disclosed this identity to other people and instead limited their transness to their private, rather than public, identity. In view of these factors and, of course, the absence of systematic historical data, the estimated prevalence of transgenderism historically can only ever be speculative.

There were a few cases of gender reassignment surgery in Europe in the early twentieth century, which generated some media coverage. Often the media coverage was sensationalist and focused on 'transformation' rather than on the construction of an identity that had long existed (Burns, 2018). A notable case that was of Lili Elbe who died after her fifth surgical procedure in 1931 (before the advent of effective antibiotics). However, the first successful case of gender reassignment surgery in the UK was that of Michael Dillon, a British physician who was assigned female sex at birth but later transitioned physically in 1946 by undergoing phalloplasty (the surgical construction of a penis). In 1951, Roberta Cowell, who was assigned male sex at birth, transitioned physically by underdoing vaginoplasty by surgery (the surgical construction of a vagina). Roberta Cowell lived as a woman until her death in 2011 at the age of 93. Both surgical procedures were performed by Sir Harold Gillies, a British surgeon who became renowned for his work in modern plastic surgery.

Although Cowell attracted some media attention during her life, she did not consistently self-identify as trans and, throughout much of her post-transition life, remained out of public view. She did write an auto-biography and shared aspects of her life with the press early on in her post-transition life, referring to herself (erroneously) as 'intersex' rather than as trans (Cowell, 1954). However, her transition (and its publicity) did not really give rise to increased public awareness or a movement to advocate for trans visibility and rights. Given the lack of visibility of trans people, many distinct labels were used to refer to their identities. The history of trans women has often been conflated with that of other groups within the LGBT umbrella category. Furthermore, as demonstrated in this volume, some trans women report initially self-identifying as gay because this is the social category with which they may initially feel that they are best aligned. This is partly attributable to dominant social representations that have historically been available to gender minorities struggling to construct an identity. The term 'trans' has of course not always existed, which essentially forced trans people to adopt the term or label that apparently corresponded to their lived experience—for some, this more readily accessible, but also stigmatised, label was that of being gay. Similarly, as Burns (2018) notes, people have identified as 'transsexual', 'transvestites' and in many other ways over the years.

It is also noteworthy that, as the LGBT rights struggle was underway in the UK and elsewhere, the approach to trans advocacy was somewhat fragmented. In 1966, the Beaumont Society was created to provide education and information about transvestism and to provide people who identified as transvestites with the opportunity to develop a social life together (Burns, 2018). Other regional groups focusing on transvestites and transsexuals began to emerge in the UK in the 1970s. In 1980, the Self-Help Association for Transsexuals (SHAFT) was created specifically to meet the needs of transsexuals (rather than transvestites). Following the collapse of SHAFT some years later, in 1988 the Gender Trust was founded to provide support to trans people but also to provide information and to advocate for trans rights. In 1992, the influential group Press For Change was created, building on the success of the Gender Trust. Its objectives were to create a network, to increase support for trans issues and to raise money to advocate for positive change for the trans community. The group was influential in social and political circles, gaining traction in the Labour Party in the 1990s. However, some of the trans groups and movements had particular foci and norms which rendered them inclusive of some but exclusive of others—for instance, Steele (2018) notes that she did not perceive a sense of belonging in the Beaumont Society, as a trans woman attracted to men. Thus, even as support groups and organisations began to emerge, not all trans women derived a sense of belonging within them and, thus, were unable to access the support that they required. It is noteworthy that the struggle for LGBT rights has not always included a focus on trans people. For instance, some forty years after its establishment, the Lesbian and Gay Foundation changed its name to the LGBT Foundation to demonstrate an inclusive approach to trans people, as well as sexual minorities. Thus, although LGBT advocacy is often understood to include advocacy for trans people, this has not always been the case.

Over the last twenty years or so, there has been important movement in the policy sphere in relation to trans people. In 2002, the Lord Chancellor's Office in the UK published its *Government Policy Concerning Transsexual People* which recognised that transsexualism was 'not a mental illness' but rather a 'widely recognised mental *condition*' and that this condition was characterised by an 'overpowering sense of different gender identity'. This marked a significant legal shift from the conceptualisation of transness as pathological. Subsequent to this publication, the Gender Recognition Act 2004 was promulgated which effectively granted legal recognition for *binary* trans people. This followed some twelve years of advocacy from Press For Change, which has been created in 1992. The Gender Recognition Act enables trans people to acquire a new birth certificate based on the gender with which they identify, provided that they meet some key criteria, namely that (1) they have received a Gender Recognition Certificate after presenting evidence to a Gender Recognition Panel, (2) that they have transitioned and been living in accordance with their identified gender for at least two years prior to receiving the Gender Recognition Certificate, and (3) that they intend to live permanently (i.e. for the rest of their lives) in accordance with their identified gender. It is not a requirement to have transitioned physically, that is, to have had hormone replacement therapy or gender reassignment surgery.

Although *prima facie* this appears to be an inclusive approach, Pearce (2018) has described the significant challenges that may be faced by trans people in convincing both medical practitioners and the Gender Recognition Panel of the authenticity of their trans identity, which can lead some to present in ways that are deemed to be conducive to an affirmative decision. This process can be difficult as there is often fear that one's identity will not be validated and approved by the Panel. Some clinicians working in the specialty of gender identity have been campaigning to change attitudes in the medical professional so that trans healthcare becomes more inclusive and more cognisant of the needs of trans patients (Lorimer, 2018).

The Equality Act 2010 was promulgated in the UK in order to reduce socio-economic inequalities by prohibiting discrimination on the basis of several 'protected characteristics' and to increase equality of opportunity for individuals with these characteristics. Crucially, 'gender reassignment' was included as one of these characteristics and the Act explicitly states that:

> A person has the protected characteristic of gender reassignment if the person is proposing to undergo, is undergoing or has undergone a process (or part of a process) for the purpose of reassigning the person's sex by changing physiological or other attributes of sex.

Although intended to protect trans people, this element of the Equality Act 2010 does not explicitly protect those trans people who are *not* 'proposing to undergo, undergoing or undergone a process (or part of a process) for the purpose of reassigning the person's sex by changing physiological or other attributes of sex'. It does not provide protection for those trans people who *present as* or *identify with* their gender identity. This has given rise to considerable debate, much of which has included overt or subtle discrimination against trans women, in particular, whose gender identity has been negated by some commentators (see Hines, 2019). In many cases, the nature of this debate has caused psychological distress to some trans people who perceive their gender identity to be negated by cisgender people. This has been discussed in more detail elsewhere (Burns, 2018; Stryker, 2017). Indeed, in the case studies presented above and the chapters that follow, we see the insidious effects of the stigmatisation of trans women on both their psychological and physical health outcomes.

It is widely acknowledged that the 2010s and, in particular the year 2015, saw the most significant shift in societal representations and understandings of trans people. Indeed, 2015 was described by the Vogue magazine as the 'year of trans visibility'. Retired Olympic gold-medal-winning athlete Caitlyn Jenner's coming out as a trans woman in April 2015 attracted a great deal of media attention and shortly afterwards she starred in the reality television series 'I am Cait'. In the same year, trans actress Laverne Cox starred in the popular Netflix series 'Orange is the New Black'. Trans people were more visible than ever before and in television and film trans characters were increasingly being played by trans actors—the tremendous successes of trans people were finally being showcased to a large audience (Burns, 2018). Yet, it must also be acknowledged that increased visibility of trans people has also uncovered the considerable prejudices that continue to bedevil our society. The ongoing debate about whether trans women should be allowed to use women's washrooms is just one example of how the identity of trans people is habitually contested by some people, with significant implications for trans people's sense of belonging, identity authenticity and psychological wellbeing.

In this brief history of trans people in the UK, there has been no mention of HIV. This reflects the conspicuous absence of trans people from HIV data and statistics (discussed below) but also from the HIV prevention campaigns which became so pervasive during the 1980s and 1990s (Jaspal & Bayley, 2020). Trans people were, and largely remain, an invisible group in the HIV epidemic in the UK, which is a key rationale for producing this volume. This represents a significant lacuna in the fields of both HIV and trans studies. As outlined in the rest of this volume, trans women face an elevated risk of HIV and trans women living with HIV an elevated risk of poor HIV outcomes than other populations.

In the era of effective ART, HIV status is not a barrier to accessing gender identity services or gender reassignment surgery (Kim, Choi, Kim, Kim, & Lee, 2015). However, trans people diagnosed in the pre-ART era and in the years immediately after the introduction of effective ART have experienced decreased access to gender reassignment surgery, because of the risks associated with performing surgery on patients with HIV/AIDS (Selzer, McAuliffe, Campbell, & Burkhalter, 1991). Furthermore, there may be other HIV-related comorbidities in this population which are deemed to render gender reassignment surgery risky. In the absence of robust scientific evidence about interactions between ART and hormone replacement therapy (an essential component of the gender transition for many trans people), there has been trepidation both from clinicians and from trans people themselves about the simultaneous use of both therapeutic inventions (one essential for the treatment of HIV and one for the successful completion of one's gender transition) (Radix, Sevelius, & Deutsch, 2016).

Clinicians who are nervous about the progression of HIV may advise their patients to interrupt hormone replacement therapy, while patients who are nervous about the impact of ART on the efficacy of hormone replacement therapy may elect to interrupt ART. Clearly, this can have a significant adverse impact on the psychological wellbeing of trans women living with HIV who wish to transition physically. Indeed, this is a significant finding from not only the EXTRA Study but also previous research into trans people living with HIV (Jaspal, Kennedy, & Tariq, 2018). However, as effective guidelines regarding the treatment of HIV in trans women emerge (e.g. British Association for Sexual Health and HIV, 2019), concerns from both clinicians and patients should be alleviated.

Trans Women and HIV: Some Statistics

The National Office for Statistics has never collected robust data on the trans population in the UK. As noted above, the Gender Recognition Act 2004 allows trans people to have their gender officially recognised and to receive a Gender Recognition Certificate. They must meet seven criteria to do so. In 2018, 4910 trans individuals had obtained a Gender Recognition Certificate (LGBT Policy Team, 2018). However, it is recognised that this captures only those individuals who have taken the step to have their gender recognised but not the broad trans population who express their gender identity in various ways. According to the Government Equalities Office (2018), it is estimated that there are between 200,000 and 500,000 trans people living in the United Kingdom. It is not known what the proportion of this broad population estimate is comprised by trans women. At the time of writing, the National Office for Statistics was examining whether and, if so, how to develop a population estimate of trans people in the UK.

Similarly, there is a shortage of robust data on the prevalence and incidence of HIV in trans populations in the UK. In an international meta-analysis of empirical data from 39 studies with a total sample size of 11,066 trans women, Baral et al. (2013) estimated a 20% HIV prevalence in trans women and concluded that trans women were 49 times more likely to be HIV-infected than the general population. However, given low rates of HIV testing and healthcare engagement in this population, undiagnosed HIV may be prevalent (Williams et al., 2016). Moreover, there are of course risk factors specific to particular cultural contexts, which means that only a country-specific prevalence study would shed light on the epidemiology of HIV in the UK.

Public Health England data show that, in 2017, 123 trans people were accessing HIV care in the UK, which represents 0.14% of all people accessing HIV care (Kirwan et al., 2019). Of the 123 patients, 88% were trans women, 56% were living in London, 62% described their ethnicity as White, and 42% were aged between 35 and 49 years. Their data suggest that trans patients are more likely to be under active psychiatric care than non-trans patients, which demonstrates the need to understand the psychosocial stressors that surround the experience of living with HIV in this population. Furthermore, in 2017, Valerie Delpech from Public Health England reported that trans patients were twice as likely to receive a late diagnosis than non-trans patients, suggesting possible barriers to accessing healthcare and, specifically, HIV testing (Jaspal, Nambiar, Delpech, & Tariq, 2018).

In order to contextualise trans people with diagnosed HIV in the epidemic in the UK, the incidence of HIV in the UK from 2004 to 2018 is presented in Fig. 1.1. It is clear that, in view of its achievements in relation to the 90-90-90 target and the advent of PrEP, the UK has seen a rapid decline in new HIV diagnoses since 2015 (O'Halloran et al., 2018). Although there has been a gradual decline in HIV incidence in

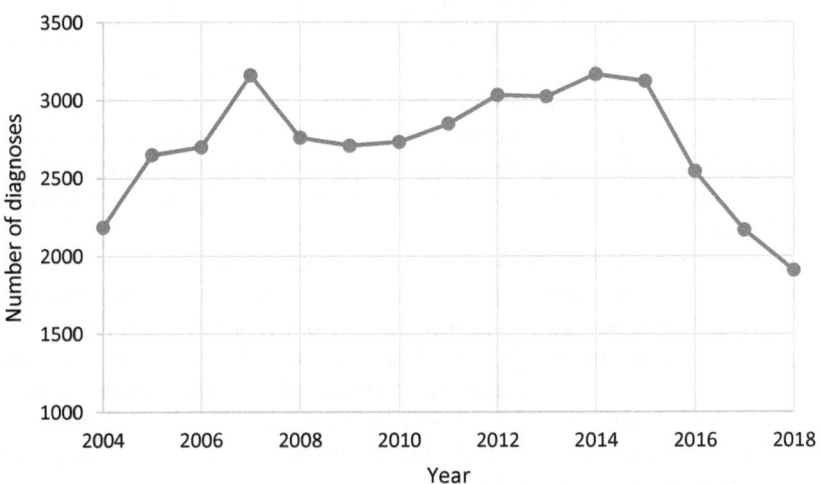

Fig. 1.1 Number of HIV diagnoses by year in the United Kingdom (2004–2018)

the UK in recent years, it is generally accepted that not all groups at risk of HIV have exhibited the same decline (Jaspal & Bayley, 2020). There is a shortage of data on HIV prevalence and incidence in trans women in the UK, which means that it is difficult to ascertain whether or not the decline clearly observable in Fig. 1.1 is also observable in trans communities. Yet, as highlighted in Chapter 3, healthcare engagement in trans women is generally low and, thus, it is likely that there is a high prevalence of undiagnosed HIV in trans women. The HIV prevention and care needs are gradually being addressed more comprehensively. In 2010, cliniQ, a community interest company for trans non-binary people's holistic well-being and sexual health, was founded. The service, which is based at 56 Dean Street in London (one of the busiest sexual health clinics in Europe), includes a multidisciplinary team of trans and cisgender healthcare professionals. Since the establishment of cliniQ, other trans-specific clinical services, such as Clinic T in Brighton, have been developed in order to meet trans people's healthcare needs in a holistic manner.

Overview of the Book

The first part of this volume focuses on trans women in context. In Chapter 2, the construction of trans identity is examined through the lenses of three theoretical frameworks: the trans coming out models; minority stress theory; and identity process theory. Identity process theory is proposed as an integrative theoretical framework within which aspects of minority stress, coming out and identity construction can be collectively examined. In this chapter, there is an examination of the factors that contribute to the construction and disruption of trans identity development.

Chapter 3 provides an overview of published research into HIV risk and HIV outcomes among trans women, focusing on the stressors that can increase the risk of poor outcomes and the coping strategies that might be enacted in the face of these stressors. Furthermore, drawing on identity process theory and the concept of structural violence from critical medical anthropology, an adapted version of the Health Adversity Risk Model is presented to shed light on responses to an HIV diagnosis among trans women in the UK.

The second part of this volume provides an overview of the findings of the EXTRA Study, which explored trans women's experiences of living with HIV in the UK. Chapter 4 explores the methodological aspects of the study, focusing on the steps taken to develop the study, the recruitment of participants and the methodologies used to generate and analyse the qualitative data which are presented in this volume. It examines the potential challenges associated with conducting research in this important area and how to attempt to overcome them.

Chapter 5 examines the multi-layered stigma faced by trans women living with HIV, which operates at distinct dimensions of human functioning, including the intrapsychic, interpersonal and intergroup levels. The chapter explores the stigmatising experiences associated with being trans and HIV-positive in a context in which both of these identity elements are minoritised and stigmatised. There is a particular focus on the implications of multi-layered stigma for identity processes.

In Chapter 6, the dual coping strategy of identity concealment and self-isolation is described in relation to trans women living with HIV. More specifically, it is shown that trans women living with HIV may struggle to resolve identity threat associated with chronic exposure to social stigma—on the basis of their trans identity and HIV-positive status—and that they attempt to cope with this by engaging in concealment and self-isolation. This chapter focuses on the ways in which this strategy may result in hypervigilance and the deprivation of social support which is crucial for effective coping.

Chapter 7 explores the interface of sex work and HIV among trans women, focusing on issues of identity management in the face of psychological stress and enforced risk associated with sex work. Furthermore, the challenges associated with sex work that are specific to trans women living with HIV are examined.

The final part and chapter of this volume draws on the Health Adversity Risk Model to provide a summary of theoretical, empirical and practical recommendations for supporting trans women living with HIV in the UK.

References

Agrawal, A. (1997). Gendered bodies: The case of the 'Third Gender' in India. *Contributions to Indian Sociology, 31*(2), 273–297. https://doi.org/10.1177/006996697031002005.

Baral, S. D., Poteat, T., Strömdahl, S., Wirtz, A. L., Guadamuz, T. E., & Beyrer, C. (2013). Worldwide burden of HIV in transgender women: A systematic review and meta-analysis. *The Lancet Infectious Diseases, 13*(3), 214–222. https://doi.org/10.1016/S1473-3099(12)70315-8.

Breakwell, G. M. (1986). *Coping with threatened identities*. London: Methuen.
British Association for Sexual Health and HIV. (2019). *BASHH recommendations for integrated sexual health services for trans, including non-binary people*. http://www.gpone.wales.nhs.uk/sitesplus/documents/1000/bashh-recommendations-for-integrated-sexual-health-services-for-trans-including-non-binary-people-2019pdf.pdf.
Burns, C. (Ed.). (2018). *Trans Britain: Our journey from the shadows*. London: Unbound.
Cowell, R. E. (1954). *Roberta Cowell's story*. London: W. Heinemann.
Government Equalities Office. (2018). *Trans people in the UK*. https://assets.publishing.service.gov.uk/government/uploads/system/uploads/attachment_data/file/721642/GEO-LGBT-factsheet.pdf.
Hines, S. (2019). The feminist frontier: On trans and feminism. *Journal of Gender Studies, 28*(2), 145–157. https://doi.org/10.1080/09589236.2017.1411791.
Jaspal, R. (2018). *Enhancing sexual health, self-identity and wellbeing among men who have sex with men: A guide for practitioners*. London: Jessica Kingsley Publishers.
Jaspal, R., & Bayley, J. (2020). *HIV and gay men: Clinical, social and psychological aspects*. London: Palgrave. https://doi.org/10.1007/978-981-15-7226-5.
Jaspal, R., & Breakwell, G. M. (Eds.). (2014). *Identity process theory: Identity, social action and social change*. Cambridge: Cambridge University Press. https://doi.org/10.1017/CBO9781139136983.
Jaspal, R., Kennedy, L., & Tariq, S. (2018). Human immunodeficiency virus and trans women: A literature review. *Transgender Health, 3*(1), 239–250. http://doi.org/10.1089/trgh.2018.0005.
Jaspal, R., & Lopes, B. (2020). Psychological wellbeing facilitates accurate HIV risk appraisal in gay and bisexual men. *Sexual Health, 17*(3), 288–295. https://doi.org/10.1071/SH19234.
Jaspal, R., Nambiar, K., Delpech, V., & Tariq, S. (2018). HIV and trans and non-binary people in the United Kingdom. *Sexually Transmitted Infections, 94*(5), 318–319. http://doi.org/10.1136/sextrans-2018-053570.
Kim, S., Choi, J., Kim, M., Kim, M., & Lee, K. (2015). Gender reassignment surgery in human immunodeficiency virus-positive patients: a report of two cases. *Archives of Plastic Surgery, 42*(6), 776–782. https://doi.org/10.5999/aps.2015.42.6.776.
Kirwan, P., Croxford, S., Kall, M., Nambiar, K., Nash, S., Ross, M., Webb, L., … Delpech, V. (2019). O22: Clinical outcomes and experiences of trans people accessing HIV care in England. *HIV Medicine, 20*(S5), 3–15. https://doi.org/10.1111/hiv.12738.

LGBT Policy Team. (2018). *Reform of the Gender Recognition Act—Government Consultation.* https://consult.education.gov.uk/government-equalities-off ice/reform-of-the-gender-recognition-act/user_uploads/gra-consultation-doc ument.pdf.

Lord Chancellor's Office. (2018). *Government Policy Concerning Transsexual People.* https://web.archive.org/web/20080511211217/http://www.dca. gov.uk/constitution/transsex/policy.htm.

Lorimer, S. (2018). 1966 and all that: The history of Charing Cross Gender Identity Clinic. In C. Burns (Ed.), *Trans Britain: our journey from the shadows* (pp. 51–67). London: Unbound.

Matsuno, E., & Budge, S. L. (2017). Non-binary/genderqueer identities: A critical review of the literature. *Current Sexual Health Reports, 9,* 116–120. https://doi.org/10.1007/s11930-017-0111-8.

Nicolazzo, Z. (2016). *Trans* in college: Transgender students' strategies for navigating campus life and the institutional politics of inclusion.* Sterling, VA: Stylus Publishing.

O'Halloran, C., Sun, S., Nash, S., Brown, A., Croxford, S., Connor, N., … Gill, O. N. (2018). *HIV in the United Kingdom: Towards Zero HIV transmissions by 2030* [2019 Report]. https://assets.publishing.service.gov.uk/govern ment/uploads/system/uploads/attachment_data/file/858559/HIV_in_the_ UK_2019_towards_zero_HIV_transmissions_by_2030.pdf.

Pearce, R. (2018). *Understanding trans health: discourse, power and possibility.* Bristol: Policy Press.

Public Health England. (2019, September 6). Trends in new HIV diagnoses and in people receiving HIV-related care in the United Kingdom: data to the end of December 2018*. *Health Protection Report, 13*(31). https://ass ets.publishing.service.gov.uk/government/uploads/system/uploads/attach ment_data/file/835084/hpr3119_hiv18-v2.pdf.

Radix, A., Sevelius, J., & Deutsch, M. B. (2016). Transgender women, hormonal therapy and HIV treatment: A comprehensive review of the literature and recommendations for best practices. *Journal of the International AIDS Society, 19*(3 Suppl 2), 20810. https://doi.org/10.7448/IAS.19.3.20810.

Seltzer, D. G., McAuliffe, J., Campbell, D. R., & Burkhalter, W. E. (1991). AIDS in the hand patient: the team approach. *Hand Clinics, 7*(3), 433–445.

Steele, C. (2018). The formative years. In C. Burns (Ed.), *Trans Britain: our journey from the shadows* (pp. 68–81). London: Unbound.

Stryker, S. (2017). *Transgender history: The roots of today's revolution* (2nd ed.). Berkeley, CA: Seal Press-Perseus Books.

Williams, H., Varney, J., Taylor, J., Fish, J., Durr, P., & Elan-Cane C. (2016). *The lesbian, gay, bisexual and trans public health outcomes framework companion document.* London: Public Health England. https://www.lon don.gov.uk/sites/default/files/LGBT%20Public%20Health%20Outcomes% 20Framework%20Companion%20Doc.pdf.

CHAPTER 2

The Construction of Trans Identity

Abstract There has been a shift in the way in which transness is conceptualised. Being trans is no longer viewed as a pathology but rather as an
identity that is assimilated and accommodated within the self-concept and
expressed in various ways to other people. In this chapter, the construction, management and protection of trans identity are outlined. First,
trans coming out models are critically evaluated. Second, minority stress
theory is discussed with reference to the stressors that trans women living
with HIV may face. Third, identity process theory from social psychology
is proposed as an integrative framework within which stressors, identity development and coping can be collectively examined. Fourth, some
empirical research into trans identity development is discussed, and the
importance of using a theoretical framework which can capture both
the multiplicity of identity and the various levels at which identity
management operates is illustrated.

Keywords Coming out · Minority stress · Identity process theory ·
Trans identity development

© The Author(s) 2020   25
R. Jaspal, *Trans Women and HIV*,
https://doi.org/10.1007/978-3-030-57545-8_2

Coming Out as Trans

Several models have been proposed for understanding the development of trans identity, focusing on the intrapsychic, interpersonal and intergroup levels of coming out. After all, coming out involves acknowledgement of one's trans identity at an individual psychological level, its disclosure to other individuals, and possible self-categorisation as a member of a group (e.g. transgender) and identification with other members of that group. The aim here is not to provide an exhaustive list of coming out models or a fine-grained analysis of the dimensions of each model but rather to provide a broad overview, which highlights some of the major strengths and weaknesses of dominant models in this area.

Bockting and Coleman (2016) developed a stage model of trans identity, building on a coming out model originally created for understanding the development of sexual identity among gay men and lesbian women. They identified the following stages: (1) pre-coming out, when they perceive a sense of difference which they attempt to conceal; (2) coming out, which involves both self-acknowledgement and disclosure to others; (3) exploration in relation to one's identity, appearance and sexual behaviour, thereby transforming shame into pride; (4) the pursuit of intimacy in relationships in one's preferred gender role; and (5) identity integration, which involves decreased preoccupation with gender categories and greater tolerance of ambiguity in relation to gender.

This model is intended to illustrate some of the steps towards the construction of a trans identity and it will undoubtedly resonate among some trans people who have had this experience. However, it cannot be considered a universal, generalisable model of coming out as trans. A key problem with this model is that there is an implicit assumption that one has to make it through each of the stages in order to reach the desired end-state of 'identity integration'. Yet, it is clear that various social and psychological factors can impact on each of these stages. For instance, in some contexts, one may come out to oneself as trans, that is, acknowledge this identity at an individual level, but find it impossible to disclose this identity to others. There may be no social or legal recognition for trans people and the individual may fear for their wellbeing if they disclose their identity to others. Furthermore, the assumption that one achieves identity integration is problematic, since the self-concept consists of multiple identities, such as ethnicity, socio-economic status, sexuality and so on. Must one's trans identity be reconciled with all of these identities in order for it to be successfully constructed?

Similarly, Devor (2004) described fourteen stages of transgender identity development in a stage-based model, consisting of: (1) abiding anxiety, (2) identity confusion about originally assigned gender and sex, (3) identity comparisons about originally assigned gender and sex, (4) discovery of transsexualism, (5) identity confusion about transsexualism, (6) identity comparisons about transsexualism, (7) tolerance of transsexual identity, (8) delay before acceptance of transsexual identity, (9) acceptance of transsexual identity, (10) delay before transition, (11) transition, (12) acceptance of post-transition gender and sex identities, (13) integration, and (14) pride. Overall, the model suggests that individuals begin the process of transgender identity development with elements of uncertainty and discomfort, followed by exploration of their emerging transgender identity, relinquishment of their previous gender identity in favour of their transgender identity, and pride in the transgender identity which is also manifested to others.

This model is considerably broader than that of Bockting and Coleman (2016) in that it incorporates the cognitive, affective and social dimensions of coming out as trans. Nevertheless, like the previous model, this one assumes that the end-state of this process is identity pride. This appears to locate the ability to derive pride in the trans individual, rather than viewing this as being heavily dependent on social context. After all, it is often very difficult to derive a sense of pride on the basis of an identity that is so heavily stigmatised in society. Similarly, the model presents the assumption that the individual will experience confusion in relation to their gender early on during the developmental process of constructing a trans identity. This too is contingent upon social context. In social contexts, in which gender diversity is acknowledged and diverse identities are supported, there is a decreased risk of identity confusion in the way suggested by the model. In other words, this model appears to reflect the specific experiences of the participant sample on which it was based, rather than reflecting the diversity of experience that trans people have in relation to their gender identity. It is, thus, unlikely to function as a satisfactory model of coming out as trans in cross-cultural settings.

Drawing on qualitative data collected from 28 transgender men and women, Clifford and Orford (2007) developed a preliminary model of transgender identity development consisting of three principal 'phases'. First, individuals develop an awareness of difference from others and, at this initial stage, attempt to manage the psychological experience of confusion about their gender, including the negative emotions provoked by this emerging awareness. Yet, they reach the conclusion that the gender identity perceived at a psychological level is at odds with their physical body. Second, they initiate the process of disclosing this emerging identity to others in their social context. They begin to communicate their confusion about their gender to other people—usually significant others, such as parents, siblings and close friends. At this stage, they may access professional assistance, such as consultation with a counsellor, psychologist or physician, but this is likely to depend partly on reactions from other people with whom they share their emerging identity. Third, they adjust to their new identity, which includes psychological and social changes. They may begin to manifest their transgender identity by referring to themselves by a name that appears to be more consistent with their gender identity, through their choice of clothing, and by initiating hormonal treatment.

In their study of 16 families, consisting of transgender and gender nonconforming youth and their cisgender caregivers, Katz-Wise et al. (2017) describe a framework consisting of six inter-related 'constructs' which culminate in gender affirmation/actualisation in transgender and gender nonconforming youth. First, it is thought that sociocultural influences and discourses shape how trans individuals and their caregivers understand gender. Second, in conjunction with biological influences (e.g. puberty), these discourses contribute to both trans identity development and family adjustment to the individual's emerging transgender identity. There is thought to be a reciprocal relationship between transgender identity development and family adjustment. Third, stigma and cisnormativity, both of which are impacted by sociocultural discourses, will also have implications for transgender identity development. Fourth, the availability of support and resources will shape transgender identity. It is noteworthy that there is a reciprocal relationship between family adjustment and the availability of support/resources. On the one hand, the availability of support/resources to the transgender individual is determined partly by family adjustment, since accepting family members tend to provide support while non-accepting family members tend not to. However, it is also true that family members require support/resources in order to be supportive of a transgender family member. In their framework, support/resources is a key construct, which is said to lead to gender affirmation/actualisation of a transgender identity.

There are several strengths of the Katz-Wise et al. (2017) framework, which require some commentary. First, though stages are implied, the model suggests that the stages are much more fluid and dynamic than in other models and also acknowledges that several pathways are bidirectional (e.g. the availability of social support). Second, the interpersonal dimension of the model appears to be grounded not only in the perspectives of transgender people (as in other models) but also in the accounts of caregivers whose reactions tend to be influential in shaping the course of transgender identity development. Third, the model does not mirror coming out models proposed in relation to gay, lesbian and bisexual people, which of course focus on the development of *sexual* identity. Rather, it proposes a model that is grounded in qualitative data from two significant sources: transgender people and their caregivers. Yet, a significant dimension of the trans experience is of course the social stigma that they encounter from hostile others. This must be incorporated into our understanding of trans identity construction.

Minority Stress

Minority Stress Theory (Meyer, 2003) has become a dominant theoretical lens for examining the relationship between experiences of discrimination due to one's sexual minority status and mental health outcomes. The theory posits that sexual minority individuals are exposed to two distinct types of stressor: distal stressors, which are external to the individual, such as heteronormativity and actual experiences of homophobia; and proximal stressors, which are internal to the individual, such as *awareness* of stigma and internalised homophobia.

These stressors relate to one's minority identity and lead to cognitions or experiences that stigmatise one's minority identity. Moreover, they are said to be unique to minority groups in that members of the heterosexual majority would not experience them; chronic because they relate to the long-standing cultural system of heteronormativity which tends not to accommodate sexual minority identities; and rooted in both social and psychological processes in that they arise from the social context but are perceived and experienced at an individual level (Meyer, 2003).

Furthermore, according to the theory, the individual develops an anticipation of negative social attitudes towards their minority identity, which reflects a form of 'hypervigilance' when anticipating, or actually engaging in, interaction with others. Collectively, exposure to distal and prox-imal stressors, in addition to the general stressors unrelated to one's sexual minority identity (e.g. poverty, life events) which can compound them, culminate in the poor mental health outcomes that are observed in research into sexual minority populations (e.g. Meyer, 2003). Research has also revealed that proximal stressors mediate the relationship between distal stressors and poor mental health, suggesting that when one inter-nalises stigma, one's risk of poor mental health increases (Hatzenbuehler, 2009).

Although the Minority Stress Theory has mainly been applied to sexual minorities, including gay, lesbian and bisexual people, it has also been adapted to trans populations in order to capture the impact of stres-sors specific to this minority group on their mental health outcomes. Breslow et al. (2015) proposed an adapted model which acknowledges (1) the impact of distal stressors, including experiences of transphobic discrimination, on depressive symptomatology, such as distress, depres-sion and anxiety; (2) the impact of proximal stressors, such as internalised transphobia, on self-construal; and (3) the causal relationship between first-hand experiences of transphobic discrimination and anticipated trans-phobia in future interactions, which can also have an adverse impact on psychological health outcomes. In their study of 552 transgender individuals, Breslow et al. (2015) found that resilience was negatively correlated with both minority stressors (e.g. transphobic discrimina-tion) and psychological distress, suggesting that this trait may perform a protective function for transgender individuals.

The minority stress perspective is useful in enhancing our under-standing the multiple layers of stigma that trans women living with HIV may face. On the one hand, they face a series of distal and proximal stressors in relation to their trans identity but, on the other hand, they experience stressors that are associated with the stigma of HIV. Collec-tively, these stressors can impinge on psychological wellbeing. Yet, neither the minority stress perspective nor the coming out models enhance our understanding of how the multiple identities of being trans and HIV-positive are constructed and integrated in the self-concept. Multiple identities and the multifarious social representations associated with them are a key focus of identity process theory.

Identity Process Theory

Throughout this volume, it is shown that transgender women are at disproportionately high risk of experiencing events and situations that can cause psychological stress. Many of the models of transgender identity development and minority stress theory suggest that these stressors contribute to the social context in which individuals attempt to construct their transgender identity. Yet, there say relatively little about *how* these stressors might shape the construction of identity.

As depicted in Fig. 2.1, identity process theory (Breakwell, 1986, 2001; Jaspal & Breakwell, 2014) provides an integrative model of how people construct their identities, the factors that can 'threaten' their identities, and how they subsequently cope with these threats. Although the theory was not developed specifically to understand identity construction, threat and coping among trans women, it does enable us to understand how minority stressors might impact identity processes and prompt particular strategies for coping.

The theory posits that individuals construct their identity by engaging in two social psychological processes: *assimilation-accommodation* and *evaluation*.

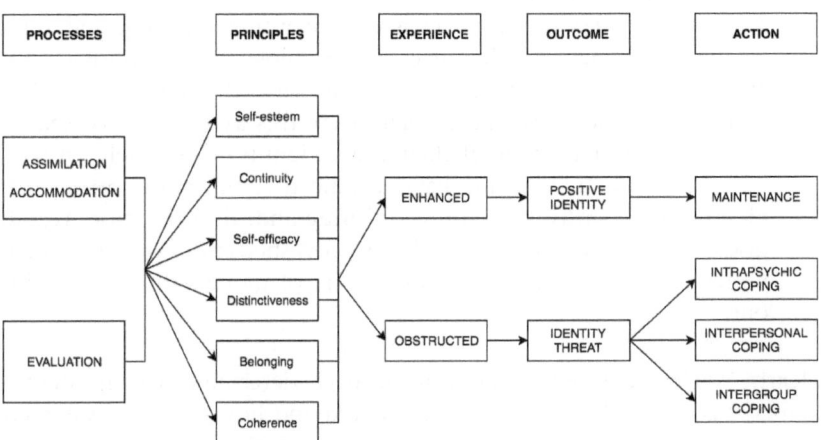

Fig. 2.1 Identity process theory (from Jaspal, 2018)

- *Assimilation-accommodation* refers to the absorption of new information (such as new identity characteristics or social representations) into identity and the creation of space for it within the identity structure. For instance, as the coming out models above note, at some point in their lives, trans people become aware that they are different from others and experience gender dysphoria but they do not automatically come as out as trans to themselves or others. Gradually, after some consideration, they may come to absorb their emerging trans identity into the self-concept (assimilation). The assimilation of this novel information may lead some trans people to question the significance of other identities in the self-concept, especially if it is deemed to be inconsistent with their trans identity. For instance, they may previously have self-identified as gay and, thus, relinquish this identity in favour of their trans identity. Furthermore, other identities, such as religion, may be seen as challenging their trans identity, especially if they have experienced rejection from religion in the past. This may lead to the abandonment of religious identity. Conversely, other identities, which are perceived as compatible with the newly assimilated trans identity, may be adopted. This can lead to changes in the identity structure in order to make room for their new trans identity (accommodation).
- *Evaluation* refers to the process of attributing meaning and value to the components of identity. For example, in transphobic societies, trans people may come to internalise the stigma appended to their trans identity and actually view this as a source of shame. They may elect to conceal their trans identity. Conversely, in societies in which trans rights have advanced significantly, one's trans identity may constitute a source of pride and, thus, be more readily disclosed to others. Crucially, this process sheds light on what determines 'identity pride' which forms part of models of trans coming out.

Clearly, social representations will in part determine which identity elements are assimilated and accommodated and how they are evaluated. The two identity processes do not function randomly, but rather they are guided by various motivational principles. These principles essentially specify the desirable end-states for identity:

- *Self-esteem* refers to personal and social worth. There is evidence that trans people may exhibit low self-esteem when they experience internalised transphobia (i.e. the uncritical acceptance of negative perceptions of trans people) and decreased social connectedness with others (Austin & Goodman, 2017). Furthermore, it is known that stigma surrounding HIV infection and those living with the condition is associated with low self-esteem among people living with HIV (Rohleder, McDermott, & Cook, 2017).
- *Self-efficacy* can be defined as the belief in one's competence and control. In a study of Chinese trans women, it was found that self-efficacy is protective against depression associated with their gender transition in that individuals felt more resourceful in relation to coping (Yang et al., 2015).
- *Distinctiveness* refers to feelings of uniqueness and differentiation from others. People do like to feel unique and different from others but this must be managed in a way that does not challenge people's sense of acceptance, inclusion and belonging in groups. Many accounts of trans people who are in the process of constructing a gender identity report feeling very different from other people in their social context (see Burns, 2018). This can be challenging for their psychological wellbeing as they can feel that they do not fit in.
- *Continuity* is essentially the psychological thread between past, present and future. The perception of loss (of identity, of relationships) is a central theme in research into people who come out as trans and their families, which amounts to a reduction of feelings of continuity (Budge, Adelson, & Howard, 2013; Norwood, 2012).
- *Coherence* refers to the perception that relevant aspects of identity are coherent and compatible. Psychological coherence is central to the accounts of many people who are constructing a trans identity. Fundamentally, trans people perceive an inconsistency with the gender assigned to them at birth and the gender with which they identify, which amounts to a lack of psychological coherence. Some of the coming out models refer to identity integration as an optimal end-state for identity. This refers to the assimilation and accommodation of trans identity in a self-concept which includes other traits, characteristics and group memberships which may or may not be deemed to be compatible with their trans identity.

It is noteworthy that this list of identity principles is not exhaustive and that it is possible that other principles are operating for particular populations. When these principles are compromised, for instance by changes in one's social context, identity is said to be threatened. Identity threat is generally aversive for psychological wellbeing. However, the degree to which one's wellbeing is compromised is determined by the nature of the threat, the number of principles curtailed by the threat, and one's ability to cope effectively.

Trans women who are socialised in contexts in which their trans identity is accepted and validated are unlikely to experience the threats to self-esteem, self-efficacy, continuity faced by those raised in non-trans affirmative contexts. Yet, as much research shows, cisgenderism is pervasive and, thus, the social context in which most trans people are exploring and constructing their gender identity is a hostile and stigmatising one (Burns, 2018; Stryker, 2017). Social representations of trans people will be negative in non-trans affirmative contexts, increasing the risk of threats to the aforementioned principles. Furthermore, personality traits, such as optimism and resilience, and access to social support are likely to reduce the impact of an adverse event (e.g. transphobia, relationship breakdown) on the identity structure, leading to a decreased risk of identity threat (Jaspal, 2018).

Identity process theory posits that people attempt to cope in response to identity threat and describes coping strategies at three distinct levels of human interdependence: *intrapsychic, interpersonal* and *intergroup.*

- *Intrapsychic strategies* function at a psychological level. Some can be regarded as deflection strategies in that they enable the individual to deny or re-conceptualise the threat or the reasons for occupying the threatening position. For instance, a trans woman may initially deny that they are trans (due to the stigma appended to this category) and instead attempt to live their life as a gay man, attributing their feelings to sexual orientation rather than to gender dysphoria. When diagnosed with HIV, an individual may actively deny their HIV status because acceptance of their reality (as an HIV-positive trans woman) may be emotionally difficult. Conversely, there are acceptance strategies that facilitate some form of cognitive re-structuring in anticipation of the threat. For instance, before coming out as trans, an individual may anticipate negative reactions from some people and pre-emptively distance himself/herself from these people to minimise the negative impact of the loss of these relationships.

- *Interpersonal strategies* aim to change the nature of relationships with others. Many are maladaptive. For instance, the threatened individual may isolate himself or herself from others or feign membership of a group or network of which they are not really a member, in order to avoid exposure to stigma. This strategy fits coherently with the denial strategy given that, while denial operates at a psychological level, passing (or feigning membership of another group) is interpersonal. A trans woman may conceal her trans identity and present as male in social contexts in which authentic self-presentation as female is deemed to be too risky for identity. Individuals may fear stigma, hostility or even violence, all of which could threaten identity. An example of a proactive interpersonal strategy is that of self-disclosure, given that this can facilitate the acquisition of support from others, which is discussed in detail in Chapter 6.
- *Intergroup strategies* aim to change the nature of our relationships with groups. Most are proactive. Individuals may join groups of like-minded others who share their predicament in order to derive social support. They may create a new social group to derive support or a pressure group to influence social representations. For instance, as noted in Chapter 1, trans-affirmative advocacy groups in the UK, such as Press for Change, served to empower trans people who were struggling to construct their gender identity in isolation. Furthermore, the creation of trans-affirmative spaces where trans people can seek effective healthcare has had a similarly empowering effect, enabling them to recalibrate their relationship with their trans identity which may have been stigmatised in other contexts. More generally, by feeling that one is not alone but rather a group member, supported by others in one's group, one is more likely to cope effectively.

Identity process theory describes a multitude of coping strategies operating at least three distinct levels—intrapsychic, interpersonal and intergroup. What determines the type of coping strategy that trans women living with HIV will use? Why might they favour one type of coping over another? Can their coping strategies be predicted? Jaspal (2018) has argued that both personality traits and the *availability* of coping strategies in a given social context will determine the threatened individual's choice of coping strategy. Furthermore, as outlined in Chapter 3, practitioners have a key role to play in signposting trans people to adaptive and effective coping strategies, as it is acknowledged that those that are most readily available to people from marginalised groups in society tend to be more individualised and less effective in the long term. It is noted in this volume that trans women living with HIV face multiple layers of social stigma in relation to various identity elements, that they appear to be less able to disclose aspects of their threatened identity to others for fear of further stigma, and that some are in precarious social and economic conditions which can further complicate the coping process. Collectively, these challenges make it more likely that they will resort to less effective coping strategies simply because the more effective ones (such as the derivation of social support) are less available to them. It is noteworthy that social representations also play a crucial role because they determine the availability and the individual's evaluation of particular coping strategies. Identity threat is by no means unusual but, given the minority status and stigma associated with trans women, threat may be more chronic and aversive for psychological wellbeing in this population.

Some Empirical Research into Trans Identity

In this chapter, relevant tenets of social psychological theories that can shed light on trans identity construction have been outlined. It is also useful to consider some of the emerging research into trans identity development and to consider this work through the lenses of these theories.

Burgess (2009) notes a series of internal and external factors, which can disrupt the construction of a positive trans identity. These include the family, schools, a lack of safe space and engagement with healthcare professionals. The experiences that one has in these contexts can decisively shape the content and value of their trans identity in that some may internalise the transphobic stigma that they encounter and, thus, experience negative emotions, such as guilt and shame in relation to it. In her telephone study of 37 individuals who had a trans-identified family member, Norwood (2012) found that trans identity could sometimes function as a family stressor depending on the meaning and value that was appended to trans identity in the family setting. These meanings and values were of course shaped by multiple factors, including dominant social representations, members of one's extended family, and friends. Family responses to trans identity in turn shape the trans individual's experience of coming out and living as a trans person within the family context. As Bockting

(2014) has noted, there is an empirical association between exposure to discrimination and psychological distress and that family support, peer support and identity pride serve as protective factors, potentially weakening the relationship between discrimination and distress. These studies suggest that there are multiple stressors operating in the lives of trans people, which could plausibly threaten various principles of identity (not least self-esteem) but that there is also a lack of social support available to trans people struggling with their identity.

As social beings, we derive a sense of self partly on the basis of how others respond to us. We must feel that our identities are recognised and 'validated' by others. Indeed, in their qualitative study of eleven trans people, Morgan and Stevens (2012) found that transgender identity recognition, acknowledgement and development and their relationships with others were important determinants of their psychological wellbeing. This demonstrates the point that identity must be 'validated' by others in order for an individual to be able to derive psychological wellbeing on the basis of this identity (see also Jaspal & Cinnirella, 2012). Furthermore, a lack of identity validation may lead people to feel threatened and engage in deflection strategies designed to hide who they 'really' are. They may attempt to conform to the norms, values and ideologies that are promoted by others among whom feelings of acceptance, inclusion and belonging are sought.

In much psychological research, there has been a greater focus on psychological adversity in trans women than on the positive emotions that they may experience during the process of constructing a trans identity. Some research has revealed a relationship between the ability to express one's gender and feelings of self-esteem and self-efficacy in the future through greater perceived resilience in the face of adversity (Singh, Hays, & Watson, 2011). Thus, it appears that, in order to derive feelings of self-esteem and self-efficacy, which are important identity principles, trans people must perceive themselves to be resilient against the minority stressors that they face. Group memberships and the derivation of social support from others are key factors that increase one's sense of resilience—indeed, when people feel connected to others, they feel more empowered and self-efficacious. They may find it easier to resolve issues that cause threats to identity. They may be able to reconstrue the meaning of threatening events and situation.

Testa, Jimenez, and Rankin (2014) examined the role of resilience in trans identity development in a survey of 3087 trans adults in the US.

They found that awareness of the existence of other trans people and first-hand engagement with other trans people were associated with increased psychological wellbeing in relation to their identity construction. More specifically, these social 'connections' were associated with decreased fearfulness, anxiety and suicidal ideation and increased comfort. This supports the notion that positive interpersonal experiences not only with cisgender people but also with other trans people are associated with increased psychological wellbeing. This reiterates the importance of support and advocacy groups for trans people. This clearly enables people to feel that they are part of a bigger community from which they can derive support if they require it.

In their study of eleven trans men, Budge, Orovecz, and Thai (2015) used grounded theory to develop a theoretical model to explain the role of positive emotion in the construction of trans identity. According to their model, trans people must have confidence to confide in, and interact with, others in order to derive 'positive reactionary interpersonal emotions', such as comfort, connection, feeling alive and so on. These positive emotions generated at an interpersonal level were then said to contribute to greater self-esteem at an intrapsychic level. Given that their study focused on trans men, it is unclear whether these results are transferable to other trans populations. The study does appear to suggest that trans individuals will encounter positive reactions to their trans identity but this is not always the case and, often, exposure to stigma from significant others, such as family and close friends, can be more impactful in creating internalised stigma. As noted later in this volume, initial adverse experiences when disclosing one's identity to others can increase the anticipation of further stigma from others, minimising the likelihood of self-disclosure and the derivation of social support in the future.

There is now some work that acknowledges the multiple identities of trans people, that is, the fact that their trans identity is not the only salient element of the self-concept but rather that they also have an ethnicity, sexual orientation, geographic identity and so on. In a study examining the intersection of multiple minority identities among trans women, namely race, sexual orientation, and socio-economic status, Budge, Thai, Tebbe, and Howard (2016) studied how distinct identity configurations may impact on mental health outcomes. Their approach is important because it addresses a concern frequently raised by trans clients in psychotherapy that only their trans identity is salient in therapeutic contexts and that other relevant issues are often overlooked. The study highlights the importance of acknowledging the multiplicity of identity among trans people seeking support, given these other identities may create a particular set of life experiences which in turn determine their mental health. Erber (2015) conducted a study of trans people living in rural settings in the US and found that, in the absence of a physical community in their social contexts, individuals made use of the Internet in order to derive a sense of community and social support and to cope with the stressors that they faced. Thus, the experiences of rural, ethnic minority, nonbinary and other minority trans people may be different. They may face particular challenges that must be understood so that they can be supported effectively.

OVERVIEW

In this chapter, three theoretical approaches to the study of trans identity construction have been outlined and critically evaluated and key research into the construction of trans identity has been described and outlined through the lenses of these theoretical approaches. While the coming out models generally propose pathways towards a positive trans identity, the minority stress model outlines the stressors that can result in poor mental health outcomes among trans people. Conversely, identity process theory specifies the social and psychological factors that can lead to threats to identity and predicts behaviours designed to restore the principled operation of identity processes. Its focus on coping provides scope for examining resilience in trans women living with HIV. As an integrative theoretical framework, identity process theory focuses on multiple levels of human interdependence—intrapsychic, interpersonal and intergroup—and acknowledges the multiplicity of identity itself. It is suggested that identity process theory ought to be used to understand how distal, proximal and other stressors operate among trans women living with HIV and, crucially, how these stressors impact the construction, management and protection of identity in this population. The theory is drawn upon in the chapters that follow.

References

Austin, A., & Goodman, R. (2017). The impact of social connectedness and internalized transphobic stigma on self-esteem among transgender and gender non-conforming adults. *Journal of Homosexuality, 64*(6), 825–841. https://doi.org/10.1080/00918369.2016.1236587.

Bockting, W. (2014). The impact of stigma on transgender identity development and mental health. In B. Kreukels, T. Steensma, & A. de Vries (Eds.), *Gender dysphoria and disorders of sex development: Focus on sexuality research*. Boston, MA: Springer.

Bockting, W., & Coleman, E. (2016). Developmental stages of the transgender coming-out process: Toward an integrated identity. In R. Ettner, S. Monstrey, & E. Coleman (Eds.), *Principles of transgender medicine and surgery* (pp. 137–158). Routledge/Taylor & Francis Group.

Breakwell, G. M. (1986). *Coping with threatened identities*. London: Methuen.

Breakwell, G. M. (2001). Social representational constraints upon identity processes. In K. Deaux & G. Philogène (Eds.), *Representations of the social: Bridging theoretical traditions* (pp. 271–284). Oxford: Blackwell.

Breslow, A. S., Brewster, M. E., Velez, B. L., Wong, S., Geiger, E., & Soderstrom, B. (2015). Resilience and collective action: Exploring buffers against minority stress for transgender individuals. *Psychology of Sexual Orientation and Gender Diversity, 2*(3), 253–265. https://doi.org/10.1037/sgd0000117.

Budge, S. L., Thai, J. L., Tebbe, E. A., & Howard, K. A. S. (2016). The intersection of race, sexual orientation, socioeconomic status, trans identity, and mental health outcomes. *The Counseling Psychologist, 44*(7), 1025–1049. https://doi.org/10.1177/0011000015609046.

Budge, S. L., Adelson, J. L., & Howard, K. A. (2013). Anxiety and depression in transgender individuals: The roles of transition status, loss, social support, and coping. *Journal of Consulting and Clinical Psychology, 81*(3), 545–557. https://doi.org/10.1037/a0031774.

Budge, S. L., Orovecz, J. J., & Thai, J. L. (2015). Trans men's positive emotions: The interaction of gender identity and emotion labels. *The Counseling Psychologist, 43*(3), 404–434. https://doi.org/10.1177/0011000014565715.

Burgess, W. C. (2009). Internal and external stress factors associated with the identity development of transgender and gender variant youth. In G. P. Mallon (Ed.), *Social work practice with transgender and gender variant youth* (2nd ed., pp. 53–64). London: Routledge.

Burns, C. (Ed.). (2018). *Trans Britain: Our journey from the shadows*. London: Unbound.

Clifford, C., & Orford, J. (2007). The experience of social power in the lives of trans people. In V. Clarke & E. Peel (Eds.), *Out in psychology: Lesbian, gay, bisexual, trans and queer perspectives* (pp. 195–216). Chichester: Wiley. https://doi.org/10.1002/9780470713099.ch10.

Devor, A. H. (2004). Witnessing and mirroring: A fourteen stage model of transsexual identity formation. *Journal of Gay & Lesbian Psychotherapy, 8*(1–2), 41–67. https://doi.org/10.1300/J236v08n01_05.

Erber, N. L. (2015). *Transgender identity development in a rural area: A multiple case study of trans-identified people* (Unpublished PhD thesis). Walden University, Minneapolis, Minnesota, USA.

Hatzenbuehler, M. L. (2009). How does sexual minority stigma "get under the skin"? A psychological mediation framework. *Psychological Bulletin, 135,* 707–730. https://doi.org/10.1037/a0016441.

Jaspal, R. (2018). *Enhancing sexual health, self-identity and wellbeing among men who have sex with men: A guide for practitioners.* London: Jessica Kingsley Publishers.

Jaspal, R., & Breakwell, G. M. (Eds.). (2014). *Identity process theory: Identity, social action and social change.* Cambridge: Cambridge University Press. https://doi.org/10.1017/CBO9781139136983.

Jaspal, R., & Cinnirella, M. (2012). The construction of ethnic identity: Insights from identity process theory. *Ethnicities, 12*(5), 503–530. https://doi.org/10.1177/1468796811432689.

Katz-Wise, S. L., Budge, S. L., Fugate, E., Flanagan, K., Touloumtzis, C., Rood, B., …, Leibowitz, S. (2017). Transactional pathways of transgender identity development in transgender and gender nonconforming youth and caregivers from the trans youth family study. *The International Journal of Transgenderism, 18*(3), 243–263. https://doi.org/10.1080/15532739.2017.1304312.

Meyer, I. H. (2003). Prejudice, social stress, and mental health in lesbian, gay, and bisexual populations: Conceptual issues and research evidence. *Psychological Bulletin, 129,* 674–697. https://doi.org/10.1037/0033-2909.129.5.674.

Morgan, S. W., & Stevens, P. E. (2012). Transgender identity development as represented by a group of transgendered adults. *Issues in Mental Health Nursing, 33*(5), 301–308. https://doi.org/10.3109/01612840.2011.653657.

Norwood, K. (2012). Transitioning meanings? Family members' communicative struggles surrounding transgender identity. *Journal of Family Communication, 12*(1), 75–92. https://doi.org/10.1080/15267431.2010.509283.

Rohleder, P., McDermott, D. T., & Cook, R. (2017). Experience of sexual self-esteem among men living with HIV. *Journal of Health Psychology, 22*(2), 176–185. https://doi.org/10.1177/1359105315597053.

Singh, A. A., Hays, D. G., & Watson, L. S. (2011). Strength in the face of adversity: Resilience strategies of transgender individuals. *Journal of Counseling & Development, 89*(1), 20–27. https://doi.org/10.1002/j.1556-6678.2011.tb00057.x.

Stryker, S. (2017). *Transgender history: The roots of today's revolution* (2nd ed.). Berkeley, CA: Seal Press-Perseus Books.

Testa, R. J., Jimenez, C. L., & Rankin, S. (S.). (2014). Risk and resilience during transgender identity development: The effects of awareness and engagement with other transgender people on affect. *Journal of Gay & Lesbian Mental Health, 18*(1), 31–46. https://doi.org/10.1080/19359705.2013.805177.

Yang, X., Wang, L., Hao, C., Gu, Y., Song, W., Wang, J., ..., Zhao, Q. (2015). Sex partnership and self-efficacy influence depression in Chinese transgender women: A cross-sectional study. *PLoS ONE, 10*(9), e0136975. https://doi.org/10.1371/journal.pone.0136975.

CHAPTER 3

HIV Stressors and Risk Factors

Abstract Trans women are an important but under-researched population in the HIV epidemic in the UK. In this chapter, some of the key empirical research into HIV among trans women is reviewed. There is a focus on individual and social factors in relation to HIV in this population. The following themes are discussed: structural violence and stressors; barriers to social support; HIV and gender transitioning; and access to and engagement with healthcare. Various lacunae in knowledge about HIV-related stressors and risk factors in trans women are outlined. It is argued that this work is necessary to reduce HIV incidence in this population, to increase their engagement in HIV care across the care continuum and to improve the health and wellbeing of trans women living with HIV. The Health Adversity Risk Model is described briefly and applied to the context of trans women living with, or at risk of, HIV.

Keywords HIV epidemic · HIV risk · Gender transitioning · Structural violence · Harm Adversity Risk Model

INTRODUCTION

Advances in antiretroviral therapy (ART) mean that life expectancy in those living with HIV is now broadly similar to that of the general population (May et al., 2014). A key aspect of the effective management

© The Author(s) 2020
R. Jaspal, *Trans Women and HIV*,
https://doi.org/10.1007/978-3-030-57545-8_3

of HIV is the HIV treatment cascade (or HIV care continuum) (Gardner, McLees, Steiner, del Rio, & Burman, 2011). According to this model of care, people must initially be tested for the virus and diagnosed, be initiated on effective ART, and achieve viral suppression, which refers to having very low levels of virus in the body. This enhances clinical outcomes, on the one hand, and reduces the risk of onward HIV transmission, on the other hand.

As indicated in Chapter 1, UNAIDS set a target of 90-90-90 for 2020, which refers to the goal of having 90% of all people living with HIV know their status; 90% of those diagnosed with HIV having sustained ART; and 90% of those on ART achieving viral suppression (UNAIDS, 2017). Although the UK has now surpassed this target, this is not equitable across all groups in the UK and trans women are thought to be a high-risk group with limited access to HIV services (UNAIDS, 2016). In short, trans women do appear to be at higher risk of acquiring HIV but also face significant challenges in accessing HIV care. This in turn may lead to poorer clinical outcomes and to increased risk of onward HIV transmission.

Although trans women are a significant population in HIV prevention and management, there is a paucity of data on the health and wellbeing of this population. Much HIV research tend to focus on men who have sex with men, some of which also includes trans women (Andrinopoulos et al. 2015; Miller, 2017). This reflects a general tendency in the literature to conflate men who have sex with men and trans women, suggesting that they are the same epidemiological population. This approach is problematic not least because it masks differences in epidemiology, access to healthcare, and the social psychological differences between these populations.

The Concept of Structural Violence

Jaspal, Kennedy, and Tariq (2018) have argued that the critical medical anthropological construct of structural violence is useful in understanding HIV risk and outcomes in trans women. They indicate that, when used in conjunction with identity process theory (see Chapter 2), it can effectively bridge the individual and structural levels of analysis in this area. In this volume, it is shown that trans women living with HIV face multiple layers of social stigma, as a result of both gender identity and HIV status, and that a theoretical approach that can capture the societal level of analysis is thus advantageous (Perez-Brumer et al., 2017).

Socio-structural approaches can complement the individualised analysis of thought and behaviour offered by identity process theory. Structural violence (Galtung, 1996) refers to violence that extends beyond the physical domain and that is 'present when human beings are being influenced so that their actual somatic and mental realizations are below their potential realizations'. Structural violence is not perpetrated by a subject but is instead 'built into the structure and shows up as unequal power and consequently unequal life chances' as a result of the uneven distribution of resources and power, and is often not perceived directly.

Structural violence originates from the field of critical medical anthropology, which draws on critical theory to consider issues of power and social inequality in ill health. There has been research and commentary focusing on the societal forces of poverty, racism, gender inequality and political violence in producing poor health outcomes in populations that face them (Bourgois, 1996; Nancy Scheper-Hughes, 1993). The concept has arisen amid critiques of more individualised approaches to risk behaviour, such as that espoused in the field of psychology (e.g. Jaspal, 2018, 2019; Jaspal & Bayley, 2020). For instance, in his research in Haiti, Russia, Rwanda and the United States, to Farmer (2004) has shown how increased vulnerability to HIV and poor access to HIV care can be explained in terms of poverty, lack of health infrastructure, unequal gender relations, discrimination and social and healthcare policy.

Therefore, it seems beneficial to draw on the concept of structural violence in analyses of HIV risk and management in marginalised groups in society, such as trans women. The concept can help shed light on the societal drivers of inequalities faced by people in this population, which may be less possible through the lens of psychological theories. More specifically, the principle of structural violence elucidates the social context in which psychological stressors can arise and negatively impact health outcomes in trans women, a group with decreased social capital, as outlined in the rest of this chapter.

Structural Violence and Stressors

Various studies suggest that trans women experience structural violence in the form of various different minority stressors and structural inequalities, which can undermine the identity principles of self-esteem, self-efficacy, continuity, distinctiveness and coherence, thereby challenging psychological wellbeing (Gordon, Austin, Krieger, White Hughto, & Reisner, 2016;

Miller, 2017). Research has shown that various HIV risk behaviours, such as engagement in condomless anal sex, sex work and substance misuse may actually constitute attempts to cope with minority stressors although they may in fact undermine health outcomes (Forbes, Clark, & Diep, 2016; Nadal, Skolnik, & Wong, 2012).

Actual, perceived and anticipated stigma in the workplace may lead some trans women to believe that they must engage in sex work in order to survive economically. Furthermore, rejection from significant others, which is widely reported by individuals who come out as trans, may lead to engagement in substance use as a means of escapism (Klein & Golub, 2016). Prejudice of this kind can severely jeopardise the self-esteem and continuity principles of identity, because trans women may be unable to derive a positive self-conception due to the stigma that they face, and valued relationships with others may change or be lost.

The co-occurrence and interaction of potentially harmful events and situations amount to stressors, as defined in minority stress theory—they are well recognised in HIV research (Singer & Clair, 2003). Stressors have the capacity to challenge the identity principles of self-esteem, continuity, self-efficacy, distinctiveness and coherence. Understanding these stressors (i.e. their nature, content and interaction with one another) can enable us to identify the opportunities and limitations in relation to both HIV prevention and strategies for engaging trans women living with HIV throughout the the care continuum. This can also enable us to understand patterns of cognition and behaviour in a population with an elevated risk of HIV infection.

Psychological and Physical Violence

The contexts of discrimination against trans women are multifarious and can include *inter alia* the family, the workplace, healthcare providers and the criminal justice system (Klein & Golub, 2016; Nadal, Davidoff, & Fujii-Doe, 2014; Ross, Law, & Bell, 2016). Furthermore, as demonstrated in Chapter 5, trans women often face multiple and intersecting forces of stigma, which can threaten identity. Trans women face both overt and covert forms of discrimination—while overt discrimination may include bullying and name-calling, covert discrimination may include 'microaggressions'. Microaggressions, in the context of race, are defined as 'brief and commonplace daily verbal, behavioral, or environmental indignities, whether intentional or unintentional' (Sue et al., 2007,

p. 271), which communicate hostility, derogation and insults towards individuals due to their minority status. For instance, it has been observed that trans women may be erroneously conflated with gay men (including, as discussed earlier, in research), which can be stigmatising and distressing because it denies the gender identity of trans women (Timmins, Rimes, & Rahman, 2017). One of the insidious effects of social stigmatisation is engagement in HIV risk behaviours, which has been observed in several groups (including trans women) (Poteat, Reisner, & Radix, 2014). These risk behaviours may constitute an attempt to deflect threats to self-esteem associated with social stigma (Crocker & Major, 2003).

There is also evidence of a high prevalence of emotional, physical and sexual abuse in trans women. In a longitudinal study, Nuttbrock, Bockting, Rosenblum, Hwahng, and Mason (2014) noted a 29–47% prevalence of psychological and physical gender-related abuse in trans women. Moreover, Miller (2017) found that trans sex workers were more likely than male sex workers to report physical abuse (see also Poteat et al., 2015). There is also a high prevalence of intimate partner violence against trans people. In one study (Langenderfer-Magruder, Whitfield, Walls, Kattari, & Ramos, 2014), it was reported that 31.1% of trans people and 20.4% of cisgender people had ever experienced intimate partner violence.

Nemoto, Bödeker, and Iwamoto (2011) conducted a study of trans women with a history of sex work and found that almost 40% of respondents had experienced childhood sexual abuse, which is known to be associated increased HIV risk (Brennan et al., 2012). Moreover, in their study of 60 trans people in Scotland, almost half of whom were trans women, Roch, Ritchie, and Morton (2010) found that 80% of the sample had experienced emotionally, physically or sexually abusive behaviour from an intimate partner.

There is now considerable evidence that trans people are at especially high risk of multiple types of violence across the life course, especially sexual violence (Stotzer, 2009). Experiences of abuse can challenge both the self-esteem and self-efficacy principles of identity—on the one hand, individuals may develop a type of cognition which leads them to believe that they are deserving of such abuse and, on the other hand, experiences of abuse can deprive the individual of feelings of control and competence since they feel powerless in the face of abuse. All of these forms of abuse are associated with increased HIV risk and poor engagement with HIV care (Jaspal, 2018). Individuals may disengage because self-care behaviours seem less appropriate in the context of decreased self-esteem and self-efficacy.

Socio-Economic Inequalities and Sex Work

Trans people are also known to face significant socio-economic inequalities compared to the general population. The National Transgender Discrimination Survey (Grant, Mottet, Tanis, Harrison, Herman, & Keisling, 2011) revealed that trans people are four times more likely than cisgender people to have a household income of less than 10,000 US Dollars per year. Moreover, they are more likely to be homeless, to experience poverty and to find it difficult to secure employment (McNeil, Bailey, Ellis, Morton, & Regan, 2012; Ross et al., 2016). Similarly, in the UK, a 2008 survey of LGBT people in Southern England revealed that only a quarter of trans respondents were in full-time employment and that they were three times more likely than non-trans respondents to report a household income of less than 10,000 UK Pounds (approximately 13,000 US Dollars) a year (Browne & Lim, 2008). The more recent Stigma Survey has shown that a third of trans people living with HIV in the UK (the majority, trans women) report food shortages and financial difficulties, although this does tend to be observable in people living with HIV more generally (Hibbert et al., 2018). Socio-economic inequalities can challenge the self-efficacy principle of identity due to the inability to achieve one's goals and the self-esteem principle due to the social stigma that is itself associated with poverty (Walker, 2014).

Both poverty and homelessness are independently associated with engagement in sex work, which in turn is related to increased HIV risk (Brennan et al., 2012). Trans women are more likely to have a history of sex work than the general population (Hoffman, 2014). A US meta-analysis showed that 24–75% of trans women have a history of sex work (Herbst et al., 2008), although in developing countries, such as Peru, the rate of sex work in trans women appears to be particularly high (Silva-Santisteban et al., 2012). Furthermore, as noted above, engagement in sex work is related to increased HIV risk possibly because of the need to meet others' sexual needs for payment (see Chapter 7). In a meta-analysis of 25 studies (Operario, Soma, & Underhill, 2008), it was shown that trans women who were sex workers were four times more likely to be living with HIV than cisgender female sex workers. This suggests that there may be other factors that compound the already high risk of HIV that is associated with engagement in sex work. Trans women who are sex workers, in particular, appear to be at especially high risk.

Mental Health and Substance Misuse

Structural violence and the stressors that are prevalent in trans people have an impact on mental health outcomes. Unresolved identity threat can lead to poor mental health outcomes, such as depression, anxiety, depersonalisation and others (Breakwell, 1986). Furthermore, some coping strategies can themselves undermine mental health outcomes. For instance, substance misuse, which is sometimes deployed as a means of escapism from psychological stress, can increase the risk of psychosis (Degenhardt, 2003). Moreover, poor mental health is associated with an increased risk of HIV acquisition and of onward transmission due to decreased self-care behaviours (Galarza-Tejada, Caballero-Hoyos, & Lira, 2017). In a survey of mental health outcomes among trans people in the UK (McNeil et al., 2012), it was found that most respondents reported current or past depression, stress or anxiety and that 54% had major or mild depression. There is a high prevalence of deliberate self-harm in, 32–52% report suicide attempts and 63% report suicidal ideation (Virupaksha, Muralidhar, & Ramakrishna, 2016). Exposure to social stigma appears to be associated with suicide attempts (Redfern, Barnes, & Chang, 2016).

There is a close relationship between mental health and substance use. Trans women are more likely to engage in substance use than the general population and this increased proneness to substance use is related to engagement in HIV risk behaviour (Hoffman, 2014). Trans women who engage in sex work may feel obliged to engage in substance misuse, on the one hand, and they may use substance to cope with the additional stressors associated with a career in sex work, on the other hand (Miller, 2017). In trans women living with HIV, substance use is also associated with onward HIV transmission given that substance use is known to impact adherence to ART in some patients, thereby compromising virological control (Garin et al., 2017). The practice of 'chemsex' (drug use in sexualised settings) is under-research in trans women but may be one way in which substance use can impact on HIV transmission risk and health and wellbeing in trans women living with HIV. Engagement in chemsex may also be related to threats to identity due to the stigma associated with the practice (self-esteem) and to the potential adverse impact for everyday functioning which can constrain one's competence and control (self-efficacy).

Deriving Social Support

Having access to social support is associated with both physical and mental wellbeing (Gibbs & Goldbach, 2015). It is also an effective coping strategy in relation to identity threat and psychological adversity (Jaspal, 2018). Given the social stigma appended to sexual minorities and trans people, trans women may experience a sense of disconnection from social in-groups and, thus, decreased access to social support. Social support can enhance resilience in trans women (Forbes et al., 2016). Consequently, decreased social support may limit the capacity of trans women to cope with adversity, which in turn may negatively impact mental and physical health (Bariola et al., 2015; Mereish & Poteat, 2015).

It has also been shown that trans people may have limited access to potentially helpful social spaces, such as HIV support groups, in part because of the stigma surrounding their transness (Westbrook & Schilt, 2013). They may feel stigmatised by others because of their gender non-conforming identity. It is noteworthy that HIV stigma can decrease access to social support among trans women living with HIV—as shown in Chapter 6, some refrain from disclosing their HIV status in order to protect themselves from stigma and rejection (Katz et al., 2013).

Social support is available only to those individuals who are willing to share their predicament, and exchange confidences, with others. In their national study of adults attending for HIV care at a UK clinic, Daskalopoulou et al. (2017) found that individuals who had not disclosed their HIV status to others reported less social support, more depressive symptomatology, less adherence to ART and less controlled HIV than those who had disclosed their status. Yet, sharing one's HIV status is possible only if a person has a trusted other, which whom to exchange confidences. In view of the low levels of social capital among trans women, as outlined in Chapter 6, they may have decreased access to social support.

There are some clear barriers to self-disclosure and the derivation of social support among trans women living with HIV. Individuals may believe that their positive diagnosis could increase stigmatising stereotypes of trans women as 'dirty' and they may themselves have internalised HIV stigma, which precludes self-disclosure (Bockting, Robinson, & Rosser, 1998). Furthermore, the association between an HIV diagnosis (and others knowing about this) and gender-based violence may also lead to trepidation about self-disclosure, since individuals may fear adverse reactions from partners and significant others (Orza et al., 2015).

HIV and Gender Transitioning

Gender transitioning is the process whereby trans people undergo change in order to live in a way that is congruent with their gender identity. Transitioning can occur within a number of spheres which may be independent of one other, e.g. social, legal and medical. It can potentially challenge the continuity principle of identity in view of the inevitable changes in interpersonal relations that occur during this process. Conversely, barriers to transitioning can be challenging for continuity because of the consequential discrepancy between the desired and actual 'selves' (Levitt & Ippolito, 2014).

Medical transitioning involves physical changes to the body through hormone therapy and/or surgical intervention. Some ART regimens are known to interact with oestrogen (one of the main hormones administered for medical transition), thereby reducing exposure to the hormone. This can adversely impact medical transitioning and induce concerns in trans patients living with HIV regarding the quality of their medical transition. Indeed, a survey of 87 trans women living with HIV in the US reports high levels of ART non-adherence as a result of concerns about drug interactions undermining the transition process (Lake, 2017), which has previously been reported by other researchers (Redfern et al., 2016). This is particularly concerning given that Wilson, Chen, Arayasirikul, Wenzel, and Raymond (2014) found that non-use of transition-related medical care among trans women (in particular, hormone therapy and breast augmentation) was associated with substance misuse, alcohol misuse and suicidal ideation. As indicated above, all of these practices are associated with increased risk of HIV acquisition/transmission. It is therefore necessary to understand perceptions of, and attitudes towards, both ART and hormone replacement therapy among trans women living with HIV so as not to compromise either their HIV treatment or their medical transition.

Body image concerns and eating disorders are prevalent in trans women (Diemer, Grant, Munn-Chernoff, Patterson, & Duncan, 2015). Weight gain has been reported with many commonly prescribed antiretroviral medications (Taramasso et al., 2017). Although there has been no empirical research into the impact of ART-related body-shape changes on trans women living with HIV, ART-related lipodystrophy (the abnormal distribution of fat that was associated with older antiretroviral agents) has been shown to cause distress and loss of self-efficacy in cisgender men living with HIV in the UK (Kelly, Langdon, & Serpell, 2009). It is important to explore body image concerns in trans women, as this may plausibly impact perceptions of HIV treatment and/or gender transitioning in this population.

There is a dearth of research into the relationship between gender confirmation surgery and HIV risk. In the case of trans women, gender confirmation surgery may involve the surgical construction of a 'neo-vagina' through a variety of procedures including penile skin inversion, partial bowel transplant and skin grafting (Dreher et al., 2018). It has been hypothesised that trans women with neovaginas may be at an increased risk of HIV acquisition due to changes in the immunological microenvironment as a result of surgery (Wansom, Guadamuz, & Vasan, 2016). Conversely, Poteat et al. (2015) argue that there are some protective factors associated with the neovagina, such as the hardening of tissue after healing. It is likely that other factors moderate the link between gender confirmation surgery and HIV risk, such as the method and quality of surgical construction, the nature and frequency of sexual intercourse and the use of lubricants. However, it is clear from the existing literature that this remains an under-researched area.

Accessing Healthcare

Trans women experience significant barriers to accessing healthcare, including HIV care (UNAIDS, 2016). This can be attributed partly to the lack of targeted services, as well as to gender discrimination and transphobic microaggressions perpetrated by healthcare professionals (Wilson et al., 2014). Nadal et al. (2012) define microaggressions as behaviours, such as misgendering (using incorrect gender pronouns), asking unnecessary intimate questions about gender and sexuality, and wilfully ignoring the existence of transphobia. They also note the adverse impact that microaggressions can have for wellbeing among trans people. It is easy to see how this can adversely affect self-esteem, and how disengagement from healthcare may in turn constitute an attempt to protect self-esteem.

The perception of poor quality interactions with healthcare professionals constitutes a significant barrier to accessing healthcare among trans patients (Kosenko, Rintamaki, Raney, & Maness, 2013). Trans patients may feel that they obtain low-quality healthcare due to a perceived lack of knowledge of trans needs among healthcare practitioners. This perception may be grounded in reality—only 13% of UK nurses surveyed felt that they were sufficiently equipped to treat transgender patients (National AIDS Trust, 2017). Stigma can adversely impact engagement with and retention in healthcare (Chollier, Tomkinson, & Philibert, 2016). An HIV diagnosis can add a further stigmatised identity element to trans gender identity, which can compound oppression and adversely affect the quality of healthcare (Bockting et al., 1998). Indeed, the 2016 UK Stigma Survey found a high prevalence of concerns in trans people (the overwhelming majority, trans women) about being treated differently by healthcare providers in a wide range of settings with substantial numbers avoiding healthcare as a result (Hibbert et al., 2018). Furthermore, lack of family and social support is also associated with disengaging from HIV care among trans women (Remien et al., 2015). Poor engagement with healthcare services can impact the HIV continuum at all points, from HIV testing to uptake and continued adherence to ART. This in turn may contribute to late diagnosis, increased morbidity and mortality, and an increased risk of onward HIV transmission.

Access to healthcare may be further compromised by low levels of HIV-related health literacy. Despite the well-documented efficacy of PrEP and post-exposure prophylaxis (PEP), two biomedical HIV prevention approaches (Fonner et al., 2016; Thomas et al., 2015), knowledge of these approaches among trans women in the UK is reported to be low. In their survey of 44 trans people testing for HIV at a sex-on-premises venue in London, Wolton, Cameron, Ross-Turner, and Suchak (2018) found that over 70% had no knowledge of PrEP or PEP, and that many expressed concerns about potential drug interactions with hormones. More generally, there is a paucity of data on the acceptability of PrEP and PEP among trans women, which means that potential barriers to uptake of these highly efficacious prevention methods are poorly understood in a group known to be at high risk of HIV acquisition (Marquez & Cahill, 2017).

Moreover, waiting lists for Gender Identity Clinics, the initial point of contact within health services for trans people wishing to transition medically, are growing (BBC, 2016). This can have important implications for the physical and psychological wellbeing of trans people, many of whom face structural violence, and some of whom are living with HIV. For example, Nambiar, Davies, Woodroffe, Pinto Sander, and Richardson

(2017) report that nearly 40% of trans people attending their specialist sexual health service in the UK self-medicate with hormones if unable to access hormones in clinical settings and may be unaware of potential drug interactions. However, it is noteworthy that the majority of those reporting non-prescribed hormone replacement therapy in that study were trans men, so there remains a need for empirical insight into trans women.

Studies suggest that trans women living with HIV are less likely to adhere to ART and less likely to achieve viral suppression than cisgender patients living with HIV (Baguso, Gay, & Lee, 2016). A recent case-notes review of 32 trans women attending a trans sexual health clinic for HIV care found that nearly a third had taken a break from their ART, and that one-fifth had a detectable HIV viral load compared to 4% among cisgender patients attending the general HIV service (Wolton et al., 2018). It is important to gain an understanding of engagement with HIV care and HIV clinical outcomes in trans women in a larger sample of trans patients in the UK. It is possible that identity concerns play a significant role in engagement with healthcare.

The Health Adversity Risk Model

The studies described in this chapter show that trans women are a key group in the HIV epidemic. This is a group at high risk of HIV acquisition, and those living with HIV are at increased risk of poor clinical outcomes associated with their infection. They appear to be less likely to access and engage with HIV care across the care continuum. In this chapter, some of the individual, interpersonal and social factors that contribute to increased risk have been briefly outlined. Both the concept of structural violence, which foregrounds some of the macro-level challenges faced by trans women living with HIV, and identity process theory provide a theoretical framework that can enhance our understanding of HIV in trans women.

In Chapter 2, it was argued that social stressors (one form of structural violence) can undermine identity processes and lead to engagement in a variety of coping strategies. This in turn can put the individual at risk of HIV and poor sexual health outcomes. The studies described in this chapter suggest that a modified version of the Health Adversity Risk Model (see Fig. 3.1) can be successfully applied to the context of HIV in trans women. More specifically, it can be hypothesised that both structural violence (e.g. transphobia, sexism, racism) and direct violence (e.g.

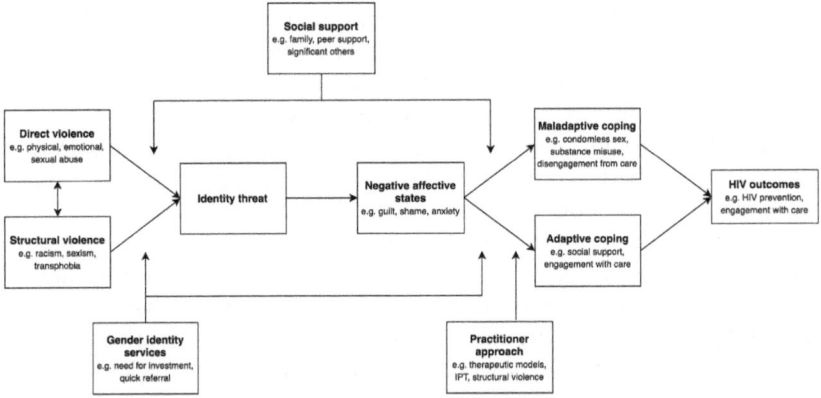

Fig. 3.1 The Health Adversity Risk Model (from Jaspal et al., 2018)

physical, sexual and emotional abuse) can threaten identity, but that this is likely to be mediated by the availability of social support and access to affirmative gender identity services, which can offer critical support in the face of gender-related adversity.

Identity process theory predicts that identity threat can result in negative affective states (e.g. guilt, shame and anxiety), which undermine psychological wellbeing. The individual in turn attempts to cope using a variety of strategies—some adaptive and others maladaptive. Coping strategies, such as condomless sex, substance misuse and disengagement from care, can increase the risk of HIV infection and decrease engagement with care among trans women living with HIV. Conversely, strategies, such as the derivation of social support and engagement with care, can prevent HIV acquisition and improve clinical outcomes among those living with HIV. The availability of social support and practitioner engagement mediates the relationship between threat and coping strategy. Therefore, it seems important to increase awareness of tenets of identity process theory and the concept of structural violence among practitioners involved in the care of trans women living with, or at risk of, HIV. Patients may be supported to adopt adaptive coping strategies and to distance themselves from those which may be maladaptive.

It is clear that this framework draws heavily on the coming out models, minority stress theory and, in particular, identity process theory to describe and predict how trans women living with HIV will cope with their diagnosis and the experience of living with the condition. Tenets of the model are drawn upon in the analysis of the EXTRA Study, which is described in Part II of this volume. However, it is suggested that this model be tested in other samples of trans women living with HIV.

Psychological and behavioural interventions for preventing HIV and for promoting better outcomes throughout the HIV care continuum could be developed on the basis of the Health Adversity Risk Model. Addressing the multiple and intersecting dimensions of structural violence, such as transphobia, sexism and racism, including within health-care settings would reduce the risk of identity threat. The increased availability of social support and a more inclusive gender identity affirming approach from practitioners would enable individuals to cope effectively before the onset of threat. An understanding of the potential risk factors for identity threat and maladaptive coping among practitioners might enable us to intervene more promptly before an adverse outcome is produced.

OVERVIEW

In this chapter, various studies of trans women living with, or at risk of, HIV have been reviewed. Most of the studies described in this chapter were conducted outside of the UK. They are described due to the paucity of UK-specific data on HIV in this population and, where appropriate, their findings are considered in the UK context. Yet, much of this existing work is valuable in enhancing our understanding of HIV in trans women. In particular, it has been shown that trans women are at risk of a multitude of minority stressors, which can undermine identity processes. Behaviours that increase the risk of poor health outcomes in trans women living with HIV may constitute coping responses in the face of psychological adversity. Maladaptive behaviours may arise in the absence of social support, which appears to be limited in its availability to trans women living with HIV. An adapted version of the Health Adversity Risk Model is proposed as a means of predicting HIV outcomes in trans women living with HIV. It is described and, in Part II, applied to data generated in the EXTRA Study. It is argued that there is great scope (and urgency) for empirical research into HIV among trans women, especially in the UK. Robust data will then enable us to develop evidence-based pathways for reducing HIV incidence in this group, for addressing inequities in the HIV care continuum, and for improving the health and wellbeing of trans women living with HIV. The EXTRA Study constitutes an attempt to begin to address the clear gap in data on trans women living with HIV in the UK.

REFERENCES

Andrinopoulos, K., Hembling, J., Guardado, M. E., de Maria Hernández, F., Nieto, A. I., & Melendez, G. (2015). Evidence of the negative effect of sexual minority stigma on HIV testing among MSM and transgender women in San Salvador, El Salvador. *AIDS and Behavior, 19*(1), 60–71. https://doi.org/10.1007/s10461-014-0813-0.

Baguso, G., Gay, C., & Lee, K. (2016). Medication adherence among transgender women living with HIV. *AIDS Care, 28*(8), 976–981. https://doi.org/10.1080/09540121.2016.1146401.

Bariola, E., Lyons, A., Leonard, W., Pitts, M., Badcock, P., & Couch, M. (2015). Demographic and psychosocial factors associated with psychological distress and resilience Among Transgender Individuals. *American Journal of Public Health, 105*(10), 2108–2116. https://doi.org/10.2105/ajph.2015.302763.

BBC. (2016). *Transgender consultation-wait 'too long'.* http://www.bbc.co.uk/news/uk-england-35605956.

Bockting, W., Robinson, B., & Rosser, B. (1998). Transgender HIV prevention: A qualitative needs assessment. *AIDS Care, 10*(4), 505–525. https://doi.org/10.1080/09540129850124028.

Bourgois, P. (1996). *In search of respect: Selling crack in El Barrio.* Cambridge: Cambridge University Press.

Breakwell, G. M. (1986). *Coping with threatened identities.* London: Methuen.

Brennan, J., Kuhns, L., Johnson, A., Belzer, M., Wilson, E., & Garofalo, R. (2012). Syndemic theory and HIV-related risk among young transgender women: The role of multiple, co-occurring health problems and social marginalization. *American Journal of Public Health, 102*(9), 1751–1757. https://doi.org/10.2105/ajph.2011.300433.

Browne, K., & Lim, J. (2008). *Count me in too. LGBT lives in Brighton & Hove.* https://cpb-eu-w2.wpmucdn.com/blogs.brighton.ac.uk/dist/2/6377/files/2019/12/CMIT_Trans_Report_Dec08.pdf.

Chollier, M., Tomkinson, C., & Philibert, P. (2016). STIs/HIV stigma and health: A short review. *Sexologies, 25*(4), e71–e75. https://doi.org/10.1016/j.sexol.2016.03.005.

Crocker, J., & Major, B. (2003). The self-protective properties of stigma: Evolution of a modern classic. *Psychological Inquiry, 14,* 232–237. https://doi.org/10.1080/1047840X.2003.9682885.

Daskalopoulou, M., Lampe, F. C., Sherr, L., Phillips, A. N., Johnson, M. A., Gilson, R., … ASTRA Study Group. (2017). Non-disclosure of HIV status and associations with psychological factors, ART Non-adherence, and viral load non-suppression among people living with HIV in the UK. *AIDS and Behavior*, *21*(1), 184–195. https://doi.org/10.1007/s10461-016-1541-4.

Degenhardt, L. (2003). The link between cannabis use and psychosis: Furthering the debate. *Psychological Medicine*, *33*(1), 3–6. https://doi.org/10.1017/S0033291702007080.

Diemer, E. W., Grant, J. D., Munn-Chernoff, M. A., Patterson, D. A., & Duncan, A. E. (2015). Gender identity, sexual orientation, and eating-related pathology in a national sample of college students. *Journal of Adolescent Health*, *57*(2), 144–149. https://doi.org/10.1016/j.jadohealth.2015.03.003.

Dreher, P. C., Edwards, D., Hager, S., Dennis, M., Belkoff, A., Mora, J., … Rumer, K. L. (2018). Complications of the neovagina in male-to-female transgender surgery: A systematic review and meta-analysis with discussion of management. *Clinical Anatomy*, *31*(2), 191–199. https://doi.org/10.1002/ca.23001.

Farmer, P. (2004). *Pathologies of power: Health, human rights, and the new war on the poor*. Berkley and Los Angeles: University of California Press.

Fonner, V. A., Dalglish, S. L., Kennedy, C. E., Baggaley, R., O'Reilly, K. R., Koechlin, F. M., … Grant, R. M. (2016). Effectiveness and safety of oral HIV preexposure prophylaxis for all populations. *AIDS*, *30*(12), 1973–1983. https://doi.org/10.1097/QAD.0000000000001145.

Forbes, C., Clark, L., & Diep, H. (2016). Positive attributes and risk behaviors in young transgender women. *Psychology of Sexual Orientation and Gender Diversity*, *3*(1), 129–134. https://doi.org/10.1037/sgd0000148.

Galarza-Tejada, D., Caballero-Hoyos, R., & Lira, L. (2017). Factors associated with HIV transmission risk in people with severe mental illness. A narrative review. *Salud Mental*, *40*(1), 29–42. 10.17711/SM.0185-3325.2017.005.

Galtung, J. (1996). Violence, peace, and peace research. *Journal of Peace Research*, *6*(3), 167–191. https://doi.org/10.11772F002234336900600301

Gardner, E. M., McLees, M. P., Steiner, J. F., del Rio, C., & Burman, W. J. (2011). The spectrum of engagement in HIV care and its relevance to test-and-treat strategies for prevention of HIV infection. *Clinical Infectious Diseases*, *52*(6), 793–800. https://doi.org/10.1093/cid/ciq243.

Garin, N., Zurita, B., Velasco, C., Feliu, A., Gutierrez, M., Masip, M., & Mangues, M. A. (2017). Prevalence and clinical impact of recreational drug consumption in people living with HIV on treatment: A cross-sectional study. *BMJ Open*, *7*(1), e014105. https://doi.org/10.1136/bmjopen-2016-014105.

Gibbs, J., & Goldbach, J. (2015). Religious conflict, sexual identity, and suicidal behaviors among LGBT young adults. *Archives of Suicide Research*, *19*(4), 472–488. https://doi.org/10.1080/13811118.2015.1004476.

Gordon, A., Austin, S., Krieger, N., White Hughto, J., & Reisner, S. (2016). "I have to constantly prove to myself, to people, that I fit the bill": Perspectives on weight and shape control behaviors among low-income, ethnically diverse young transgender women. *Social Science and Medicine, 165,* 141–149. https://doi.org/10.1016/j.socscimed.2016.07.038.

Grant, J. M., Mottet, L. A., Tanis, J., Harrison, J., Herman, J. L., & Keisling, M. (2011). *Injustice at every turn: A report of the National Transgender Discrimination Survey.* Washington, DC: National Center for Transgender Equality and National Gay and Lesbian Task Force. www.thetaskforce.org/downloads/reports/reports/ntds_full.pdf.

Herbst, J. H., Jacobs, E. D, Finlayson, T. J., McKleroy, V. S., Neumann, M. S., & Crepaz, N. (2008). HIV/AIDS Prevention Research Synthesis Team. Estimating HIV prevalence and risk behaviors of transgender persons in the United States: A systematic review. *AIDS and Behavior, 12*(1), 1–17. https://doi.org/10.1007/s10461-007-9299-3.

Hibbert, M., Wolton, A., Crenna-Jennings, W., Benton, L., Kirwan, P., Lut, I., ... Delpech, V. (2018). Experiences of stigma and discrimination in social and healthcare settings among trans people living with HIV in the UK. *AIDS Care, 30*(7), 836–843. https://doi.org/10.1080/09540121.2018.1436687.

Hoffman, B. R. (2014). The interaction of drug use, sex work and HIV among transgender women. *Substance Use and Misuse, 49*(8), 1049–1053. https://doi.org/10.3109/10826084.2013.855787.

Jaspal, R. (2018). *Enhancing sexual health, self-identity and wellbeing among men who have sex with men: A guide for practitioners.* London: Jessica Kingsley Publishers.

Jaspal, R. (2019). *The social psychology of gay men.* London: Palgrave. https://doi.org/10.1007/978-3-030-27057-5.

Jaspal, R., & Bayley, J. (2020). *HIV and gay men: Clinical, social and psychological aspects.* London: Palgrave. https://doi.org/10.1007/978-981-15-7226-5.

Jaspal, R., Kennedy, L., & Tariq, S. (2018). Human immunodeficiency virus and trans women: A literature review. *Transgender Health, 3*(1), 239–250. https://doi.org/10.1089/trgh.2018.0005.

Katz, I., Ryu, A., Onuegbu, A., Psaros, C., Weiser, S., Bangsberg, D., & Tsai, A. (2013). Impact of HIV-related stigma on treatment adherence: Systematic review and meta-synthesis. *Journal of the International AIDS Society, 16*(3, Suppl. 2), 18640. https://doi.org/10.7448/ias.16.3.18640.

Kelly, J., Langdon, D., & Serpell, L. (2009). The phenomenology of body image in men living with HIV. *AIDS Care, 21*(12), 1560–1567. https://doi.org/10.1080/09540120902923014.

Klein, A., & Golub, S. A. (2016). Family rejection as a predictor of suicide attempts and substance misuse among transgender and gender nonconfirming adults. *LGBT Health,* 3(3), 193–199. https://doi.org/10.1089/lgbt.2015. 0111.

Kosenko, K., Rintamaki, L., Raney, S., & Maness, K. (2013). Transgender patient perceptions of stigma in health care contexts. *Medical Care, 51,* 819–822. https://doi.org/10.1097/MLR.0b013e31829fa90d.

Lake, J. (2017). *High levels of treatment non-adherence due to concerns for interactions between antiretroviral therapy and feminizing hormones among transgender women in Los Angeles, CA.* Paper presented at the 9th International AIDS Society Conference on HIV Science, July 24.

Langenderfer-Magruder, L., Whitfield, D. L., Walls, N. E., Kattari, S. K., & Ramos, D. (2014). Experiences of intimate partner violence and subsequent police reporting among lesbian, gay, bisexual, transgender, and queer adults in Colorado: Comparing rates of cisgender and transgender victimization. *Journal of Interpersonal Violence, 31*(5), 855–871. https://doi.org/10.1177/0886260514556767.

Levitt, H. M., & Ippolito, M. R. (2014). Being transgender: The experience of transgender identity development. *Journal of Homosexuality, 61*(12), 1727–1758. https://doi.org/10.1080/00918369.2014.951262.

Marquez, S., & Cahill, S. (2017). *Transgender women and pre-exposure prophylaxis for HIV prevention: What we know and what we still need to know.* http://www.avac.org/sites/default/files/resource-files/PrEP_Transgender_Women_NCIHC.pdf.

May, M. T., Gompels, M., Delpech, V., Porter, K., Orkin, C., Kegg, S., … UK Collaborative HIV Cohort (UK CHIC) Study. (2014). Impact on life expectancy of HIV-1 positive individuals of CD4+ cell count and viral load response to antiretroviral therapy. *AIDS, 28*(8), 1193–1202. https://doi.org/10.1097/QAD.0000000000000243.

McNeil, J., Bailey, L., Ellis, S., Morton, J., & Regan, M. (2012). *Trans mental health and emotional wellbeing study 2012.* Scottish Transgender Alliance. http://www.scottishtrans.org/wp-content/uploads/2013/03/trans_mh_study.pdf.

Mereish, E., & Poteat, V. (2015). A relational model of sexual minority mental and physical health: The negative effects of shame on relationships, loneliness, and health. *Journal of Counseling Psychology, 62*(3), 425–437. https://doi.org/10.1037/cou0000088.

Miller, W. (2017). *Contextual factors that contribute to increased risk of HIV among transgender and MSM sex workers and recommendations for service delivery.* Dissertation Abstracts International: Section B: The Sciences And Engineering. 77(11-B):E.

Nadal, K., Davidoff, K., & Fujii-Doe, W. (2014). Transgender women and the sex work industry: Roots in systemic, institutional, and interpersonal discrimination. *Journal of Trauma & Dissociation, 15*(2), 169–183. https://doi.org/10.1080/15299732.2014.867572.

Nadal, K., Skolnik, A., & Wong, Y. (2012). Interpersonal and systemic microaggressions toward transgender people: Implications for counseling. *Journal of LGBT Issues in Counseling, 6*(1), 55–82. https://doi.org/10.1080/15538605.2012.648583.

Nambiar, K., Davies, J., Woodroffe, T., Pinto Sander, N., & Richardson, D. (2017). Beyond sexual health: Identifying healthcare needs of trans and gender variant people in a specialist clinic service. *Sexually Transmitted Infections, 93*(A10). http://doi.org/10.1136/sextrans-2017-053232.27.

National AIDS Trust. (2017). *Trans* people and HIV*. London. http://www.nat.org.uk/sites/default/files/publications/NAT%20Trans%20Evidence%20Review%20V3%20Digital.pdf.

Nemoto, T., Bödeker, B., & Iwamoto, M. (2011). Social support, exposure to violence and transphobia, and correlates of depression among male-to-female transgender women with a history of sex work. *American Journal of Public Health, 101*(10), 1980–1988. https://doi.org/10.2105/AJPH.2010.197285.

Nuttbrock, L., Bockting, W., Rosenblum, A., Hwahng, S., & Mason, M. (2014). Gender abuse, depressive symptoms, and substance use among transgender women: A 3-year prospective study. *American Journal of Public Health, 104*(11), 2199–2206. https://doi.org/10.2105/AJPH.2014.302106.

Operario, D., Soma, T., & Underhill, K. (2008). Sex work and HIV status among transgender women: Systematic review and meta-analysis. *JAIDS Journal of Acquired Immune Deficiency Syndromes, 48*(1), 97–103. https://doi.org/10.1097/qai.0b013e31816e3971.

Orza, L., Bewley, S., Chung, C., Crone, E. T., Nagadya, H., Vazquez, M., Welbourn, A. (2015). "Violence. Enough already": Findings from a Global Participatory Survey Among Women Living with HIV. *Journal of the International AIDS Society, 18*(6, Suppl. 5), 20285. https://doi.org/10.7448/ias.18.6.20285.

Perez-Brumer, A. G., Reisner, S. L., McLean, S. A., Silva-Santisteban, A., Huerta, L., Mayer, K. H., … Lama, J. R. (2017). Leveraging social capital: Multilevel stigma, associated HIV vulnerabilities, and social resilience strategies among transgender women in Lima, Peru. *Journal of the International AIDS Society, 20*(1), 21462. https://doi.org/10.7448/IAS.20.1.21462.

Poteat, T., Reisner, S. L., & Radix, A. (2014). HIV epidemics among transgender women. *Current Opinion in HIV and AIDS, 9*(2), 168–173. https://doi.org/10.1097/COH.0000000000000030.

Poteat, T., Wirtz, A. L., Radix, A., Borquez, A., Silva-Santisteban, A., Deutsch, M. B., … Operario, D. (2015). HIV risk and preventive interventions in transgender women sex workers. *Lancet (London, England)*, *385*(9964), 274–286. https://doi.org/10.1016/S0140-6736(14)60833-3.

Redfern, J., Barnes, A., & Chang, J. (2016). Psychosocial, HIV, and health care management issues impacting transgender individuals. *American Journal of Orthopsychiatry, 86*(4), 366–372. https://doi.org/10.1037/ort0000190.

Remien, R. H., Bauman, L. J., Mantell, J. E., Tsoi, B., Lopez-Rios, J., Chhabra, R., … Warne, P. (2015). Barriers and facilitators to engagement of vulnerable populations in HIV primary care in New York City. *Journal of acquired immune deficiency syndromes, 69* (0 1, Suppl. 1), S16–S24. https://doi.org/10.1097/QAI.0000000000000577.

Roch, A., Ritchie, G., & Morton, J. (2010). *Out of sight, out of mind? Transgender people's experiences of domestic abuse.* Scottish Transgender Alliance. http://www.scottishtrans.org/wp-content/uploads/2013/03/trans_domestic_abuse.pdf.

Ross, K., Law, M., & Bell, A. (2016). Exploring healthcare experiences of transgender individuals. *Transgender Health, 1*(1), 238–249. https://doi.org/10.1089/trgh.2016.0021.

Scheper-Hughes, N. (1993). *Death without weeping: The violence of everyday life in Brazil.* Berkeley and Los Angeles: University of California Press.

Silva-Santisteban, A., Raymond, H. F., Salazar, X., Villayzan, J., Leon, S., McFarland, W., & Caceres, C. F. (2012). Understanding the HIV/AIDS epidemic in transgender women of Lima, Peru: Results from a sero-epidemiologic study using respondent driven sampling. *AIDS and Behaviour, 16*(4), 872–881. https://doi.org/10.1007/s10461-011-0053-5.

Singer, M., & Clair, S. (2003). Syndemics and public health: Reconceptualising disease in bio-social context. *Medical Anthropology Quarterly, 17*(4), 423–441. https://doi.org/10.1525/maq.2003.17.4.423.

Stotzer, R. L. (2009). Violence against transgender people: A review of United States data. *Aggression and Violent Behaviour, 14*(3), 170–179. https://doi.org/10.1016/j.avb.2009.01.006.

Sue, D. W., Capodilupo, C. M., Torino, G. C., Bucceri, J. M., Holder, A. M. B., Nadal, K. L., & Esquilin, M. (2007). Racial microaggressions in everyday life: Implications for clinical practice. *American Psychologist, 62*(4), 271–286. https://doi.org/10.1037/0003-066X.62.4.271.

Taramasso, L., Ricci, E., Menzaghi, B., Orofino, G., Passerini, S., Madeddu, G., … CISAI Study Group. (2017). Weight gain: A possible side effect of all antiretrovirals. *Open Forum Infectious Diseases, 4*(4), ofx239. https://doi.org/10.1093/ofid/ofx239.

Thomas, R., Galanakis, C., Vézina, S., Longpré, D., Boissonnault, M., Huchet, E., … Machouf, N. (2015). Adherence to Post-Exposure Prophylaxis (PEP) and incidence of HIV seroconversion in a major North American Cohort. *PloS One, 10*(11), e0142534. https://doi.org/10.1371/journal.pone.0142534.

Timmins, L., Rimes, K., & Rahman, Q. (2017). Minority stressors and psychological distress in transgender individuals. *Psychology of Sexual Orientation and Gender Diversity, 4*(3), 328–340. https://doi.org/10.1037/sgd0000237.

UNAIDS (2016). Prevention gap report. https://www.unaids.org/sites/def ault/files/media_asset/2016-prevention-gap-report_en.pdf

UNAIDS (2017). Ending AIDS: Progress towards the 90-90-90-targets. https://www.unaids.org/sites/default/files/media_asset/Global_AIDS_u pdate_2017_en.pdf

Virupaksha, H., Muralidhar, D., & Ramakrishna, J. (2016). Suicide and suicidal behavior among transgender persons. *Indian Journal of Psychological Medicine, 38*(6), 505–509. https://doi.org/10.4103/0253-7176.194908.

Walker, R. (2014). *The shame of poverty.* Oxford: Oxford University Press. https://doi.org/10.1093/acprof:oso/9780199684823.001.0001.

Wansom, T., Guadamuz, T., & Vasan, S. (2016). Transgender populations and HIV: Unique risks, challenges and opportunities. *Journal of Virus Eradication, 2*(2), 87–93.

Westbrook, L., & Schilt, K. (2013). Doing gender, determining gender: Transgender people, gender panics, and the maintenance of the sex/gender/sexuality system. *Gender & Society, 28*(1), 32–57. https://doi. org/10.1177/0891243213503203.

Wilson, E., Chen, Y., Arayasirikul, S., Wenzel, C., & Raymond, H. (2014). Connecting the dots: Examining transgender women's utilization of transition-related medical care and associations with mental health, substance use, and HIV. *Journal of Urban Health, 92*(1), 182–192. https://doi.org/10.1007/s11524-014-9921-4.

Wolton, A. J., Cameron, R., Ross-Turner, M., & Suchak, T. (2018). Trans:Mission: A community-led HIV testing initiative for trans people and their partners at a London sex-on-premises venue. *HIV Nursing, 18*(2), 24–29.

PART II

Trans Women Living with HIV in the UK

CHAPTER 4

Researching HIV and Trans Women

Abstract Conducting research should be an exciting and challenging process. If it were not, many of us probably would not carry out the research in the first place. Potential challenges include formulating high-quality research questions, gaining access to participants and data, developing an effective coding scheme, selecting the most appropriate research method, conducting the analysis and disseminating the results effectively to stakeholders. In this chapter, each of these essential steps is outlined and discussed in relation to the EXTRA (EXperiences of TRAns women living with HIV) Study in the UK. The methodological aspects of the EXTRA Study are described, and a rationale for key methodological decisions is provided.

Keywords Thematic analysis · Interview research · Participant recruitment · Rapport · Ethics

FOUR KEY FACTORS IN QUALITATIVE RESEARCH

In this section, four key factors that should be considered during the research process are outlined. These include developing the research questions that will be addressed in the project; gaining access to participants and generating data for analysis; and effective engagement with research participants. These factors are examined in relation to the EXTRA Study.

© The Author(s) 2020   67
R. Jaspal, *Trans Women and HIV*,
https://doi.org/10.1007/978-3-030-57545-8_4

Developing the Research Questions

As indicated in Chapter 3, globally trans women appear to be at higher risk of acquiring HIV and of experiencing poorer HIV outcomes than other groups in society. However, when the possibility of exploring the experiences of trans women living with HIV was first considered, it was not entirely clear whether trans women in the UK were at especially high risk of HIV or even how many trans women were living with HIV in the UK. In short, there were no reliable epidemiological data on the prevalence or incidence of HIV in trans people. On the one hand, all of the evidence from global studies suggested that this was an important question to be posing in HIV research but, on the other hand, it seemed difficult to present a case for exploring the experience of living with HIV in this population in the absence of robust data from the UK context. As indicated in Part II of this volume, the emerging data in the UK do suggest that trans women are a key population in the HIV epidemic. Furthermore, in order to promote effective healthcare for all sections of society, it is important to investigate their experiences of healthcare irrespective of disease prevalence within this group (see Jaspal, in press).

The first step was to explore the literature on HIV in transgender communities, which resulted in a narrative literature review (Jaspal, Kennedy, & Tariq, 2018). One of the most important observations made in the literature review was that much of the existing research had, to some extent, captured the experiences of trans women living with HIV but that these data were frequently conflated with those from men who have sex with men. In other words, it was being assumed that trans women were not sufficiently different from men who have sex with men and by extension that their experiences were likely to be similar. Thus, many researchers simply did not disaggregate the data from these two separate groups. It seemed important to examine the first-hand accounts of trans women, in particular, in relation to their experiences of living with HIV. Second, the review suggested that stigma and discrimination were significant themes throughout the existing literature on this population, and that trans women were experiencing these challenges in relation to various identities: gender, appearance, HIV status. This too suggested that there was merit in examining the experiences of this population, as well as the specific role of stigma and discrimination in shaping them. Third, sex work emerged as an important focus in previous research into trans women who are more likely to engage in this practice than other populations, mainly due to socio-economic barriers and exclusion from other occupational possibilities. Through this process, the following research questions were identified:

- How do trans women living with HIV experience their diagnosis and the stressors associated with the condition?
- How do they perceive and manage HIV disclosure?
- How does the experience of living with HIV shape identity and psychological wellbeing among trans women?

Access to Participants and Data

An editorial in *Sexually Transmitted Infections* focusing on the need for robust empirical research into HIV in trans communities (Jaspal, Nambiar, Delpech, & Tariq, 2018) began with the following quote from Laverne Cox who spoke at the Social Good Summit in 2015:

> What message are we sending to young people who are trans or gender nonconforming when we don't even count them? We suggest their identities don't even matter.

These inspiring words highlight the power of research to promote positive social change. Yet, they also beg the question as to why trans people are so under-represented in existing research and, more importantly, what researchers can do to increase their representation. As the EXTRA Study was being planned, there was also some consideration of the potential barriers to research experienced by trans communities. Given the commonplace observations that trans communities were invisible, 'hard to reach' and generally disengaged from mainstream healthcare services, the prospect of doing research with this community seemed bleak. Thus, a great deal of effort went into raising the profile of the EXTRA Study and publicising its aims and the potential impact of its findings to various stakeholders—most importantly, trans women living with HIV in the UK. A three-pronged recruitment strategy was developed. The aim here is to describe the recruitment strategy and to consider its advantages and limitations in order to optimise future research in this important area.

First, there was a press release[1] at De Montfort University (Leicester, UK) where the principal investigator was based at the time of the study. The press release was far-reaching as it was published on the university website and on social media, and reproduced by various high-profile organisations in the HIV sector, such as the Terrence Higgins Trust. This approach was successful in that the researcher was subsequently approached by prospective participants on social media who were able to learn more about the project, discuss the possibility of participating in it, and take an informed decision about whether or not to participate. However, this approach did entail an element of sampling bias in that only those trans women who had access to the Internet and who were active on social media were being engaged. Perhaps those experiencing isolation and social, psychological and economic stressors (such as those illustrated in Chapter 1) were less likely to become aware of the study and to participate in it.

Second, various organisations and charities whose remit included the health and wellbeing of trans communities were approached for assistance with recruitment. It must be said that there were mixed responses to the project. Many individuals within these organisations were very supportive of the project and immediately saw its merit and value, recognising the desperate need for robust data on trans communities. They made every effort to support the recruitment of potential participants who could share their experiences of living with HIV. However, it became clear that many of the organisations had only a limited number of clients and service users from the trans community and, thus, their capacity to assist was similarly limited. A very small minority of individuals (who actually did have the capacity to assist with recruitment) approached the project with trepidation and, in particular, questioned the legitimacy of a project on trans women being led by an out-group (cisgender) researcher. Indeed, it has been shown that there can be suspicion towards research led by out-groups and that this is one of the reasons underpinning non-participation (e.g. Thompson et al., 1996). Yet, it is also clear that the 'curious outsider' approach adopted by an out-group researcher can also be advantageous for the research process because an out-group researcher may enquire about issues about which an in-group researcher may make

[1] https://www.dmu.ac.uk/about-dmu/news/2017/september/academics-launch-first-study-of-trans-women-living-with-hiv.aspx. Accessed on 21 May 2020.

assumptions (Coloma, 2008). Furthermore, once trust is established, participants may value the opportunity to explore aspects of their lived experience with an interested outsider. This was certainly the stated experience of the interviewees in the EXTRA Study. Nevertheless, the fact that the researcher was not an in-group member did result in some difficulty in recruiting participants.

Third, a snowball sampling strategy was attempted, as it was assumed that trans women living with HIV might be able to signpost potentially interested others to the study if they met the eligibility criteria. This too was somewhat challenging because, as discussed later in Chapter 6, very few of the trans interviewees were open about their HIV status to others in their social circle and many actively concealed their serostatus. They expressed immense trepidation about disclosing their HIV status to others and, though some suspected that a friend may be living with HIV, felt uneasy about broaching the issue with them. Furthermore, even those who were open about their HIV status reported knowing few other women who had disclosed their HIV status to them. Indeed, as Ellard-Gray, Jeffrey, Choubak, and Crann (2015) note in their review article, challenges in participant recruitment may be attributed to participant mistrust of the research process, and perceived risks associated with participation, such as involuntary disclosure of one's HIV status. While it was assumed, on the basis of research with other minority populations, that snowball sampling might constitute an effective participant recruitment strategy, it actually proved to be inadequate.

For future research in this area, it is suggested that a multi-pronged recruitment approach be utilised. None of the approaches above was perfect but each generated some interest in the study and, collectively, they facilitated access to an adequate sample of participants for the study to take place. The aforementioned challenges associated with participant recruitment should be considered in advance and robust strategies for mitigating them should be developed. It would be advantageous to work in close collaboration with the National Health Service (NHS) as this would ensure that a larger number of eligible participants are reached, enabling them to learn more about the study and the value of their contribution and to take an informed decision about participation.

Engagement with Participants

It is important to establish rapport with participants in a qualitative interview study, primarily because it will be difficult for them to share intimate aspects of their lives and psychological worlds with the interviewer in the absence of such rapport. The term 'rapport' itself can be understood in a number of ways. Put simply, the participant must feel at ease with the interviewer who should be clearly accepting of the participant's identity, genuinely interested and non-judgemental. As noted above, the fact that the project was being led by a cisgender man did present some challenges in relation to participant recruitment. Most participants reported experiences of transphobia, including from gay men. However, in each of the interviews, there was an excellent sense of rapport between the interviewer and interviewee, which resulted in a rich dataset.

There is a debate about insider and outsider dynamics in research (see Bennett, 1996; Jaspal, 2009; Siraj, 2012), which need not be repeated here. However, it is worth noting that being an in-group member is by no means a prerequisite, or even an advantage, for conducting research into a particular group. On the contrary, it could be argued that 'knowing an experience requires more than simply having it; knowing implies being able to identify, describe and explain' (Fay, 1996, p. 20). Indeed, in the context of the EXTRA Study, the researcher's out-group identity (as an ethnic minority cisgender gay man) was actually advantageous because it enabled the interviewees to discuss their experiences with an empathic outsider who nevertheless had an understanding of being a minority.

It is noteworthy that there were some elements of shared experience—most participants reported attempting to live as gay men before deciding to transition and reported the social and psychological challenges, which they experienced in attempting to assimilate and accommodate a gay identity prior to transitioning. Furthermore, the interviewer and participants converged somewhat in their shared experiences of 'otherness' and stigma during their lives—while the participants described these experiences in relation to their trans identities, the interviewer shared his experiences in relation to his ethnicity and sexual orientation. These were just some of the issues that created a sense of shared experience, understanding and empathy. Yet, there were of course clear divergences in experience, which resulted not in a breakdown in rapport, as some have erroneously anticipated (see Horowitz, 1986), but rather in participants' commitment to explain their experiences in a detailed manner that would resonate with the researcher. This was extremely advantageous because it generated detailed, rich and insightful accounts of participants' identities and lived experience in relation to their HIV infection. The experience of conducting the interviews demonstrated unequivocally the central importance of successful rapport-building between researcher and participant.

Although rapport is very important, it is also crucial that there are clear 'boundaries' between the interviewer and interviewee. It has been noted that the interviewer did share some of his own experiences—sometimes in response to a direct question from participants and sometimes as a spontaneous response to a comment made by the participant. In all cases, the interviewer should be empathic towards the participant but not cross the 'boundary' of becoming a therapist or advisor. An interview characterised by rapport between interviewer and interviewee may be experienced by the participant as a conversation (see also Jaspal, 2020). This is not necessarily a shortcoming but can introduce the risk that the participant asks the interviewer for advice or guidance. This should be managed effectively and responsibly, and it should be made clear that the interviewer is there to learn, not to advise or guide. Yet, the interviewer does also have an ethical responsibility to signpost the interviewee to possible support and counselling services that may be of benefit. This would usually occur during the debrief session after the study.

Maintaining transparency and honesty with interview participants is very important from an ethical perspective and is also central to establishing and maintaining rapport with them. During the course of research, participants may legitimately wonder about the researcher's personal motivations for conducting the research, especially if relevant aspects of the researcher's identity (e.g. gender, HIV status) differ from those of the participants. Some participants explicitly ask about these identity elements. In the context of the EXTRA Study, some interviewees did wonder why an HIV-negative cisgender gay male researcher was interested in studying the experiences of trans women living with HIV. This was by no means a barrier to participation but a genuine enquiry from research participants. Yet, they were aware of the interviewer's track record in research into HIV in a variety of populations—men who have sex with men, ethnic minorities, people living with long-term HIV and others. The interviewer made explicit his deep appreciation of diversity in all its guises, including gender diversity, and his desire to know more about trans women living with HIV. Interestingly, one of the participants also enquired about the interviewer's religious identity, noting that he had conducted research into both antisemitism *and* Islamophobia. Was he Jewish or Muslim? His response was unequivocal: 'Discrimination of any kind is abhorrent. It must be investigated. Solutions must be found'. This clarified the researcher's position that we all have a collective responsibility to use our skills and available tools to understand societal challenges and to attempt to address them. It is quite possible that participants' knowledge of the researcher's identity aspects had an impact on their responses and self-presentation during the interviews.

All of the interviewees were asked about their own motivations for participating in the EXTRA Study. The vast majority indicated explicitly that they wished to raise awareness of trans healthcare and, specifically, of the challenges faced by trans women living with HIV in order to facilitate improvements in healthcare. As described in the remaining chapters in Part II, several interviewees described first-hand adverse experiences in relation to their own healthcare. In view of the adverse psychological impact of these experiences, they derived great satisfaction from the knowledge that this research might inform the development of guidance for practitioners involved in the care of trans people living with HIV. Participants were informed that, at the time of the study, guidance was being developed for the provision of effective sexual healthcare for trans and gender non-binary patients (British Association for Sexual Health and HIV, 2019). By discussing their own experiences, many believed that they would be 'doing their bit' to improve the lives of trans women. Indeed, a principal objective of this volume is to ensure that both practitioners and policymakers benefit from the insights provided and this was made clear to interviewees at the outset.

An additional issue of note concerns the potential power relations between researcher and participant. Participants may sometimes attribute the category of 'expert' to the researcher because of the researcher's educational background, status as a researcher and academic knowledge of the research area. This can sometimes limit the scope of the research, as the interviewee may assume that the researcher is already aware of issues that actually require detailed discussion in an empirical context and, consequently, they may not provide sufficient depth in their responses. Furthermore, the interviewee may be hesitant about providing 'wrong' answers to questions when actually there are no wrong answers. Conversely, they may be keen to provide socially desirable responses to questions posed by the interviewer. In a few interviews, participants qualified their responses with statements, such as 'you must already know that' or 'I won't go into detail about that because you must hear that a lot'. These assumptions about the interviewer's prior knowledge represented an impediment to the generation of a rich dataset that might subsequently lend itself to qualitative analysis. It was necessary to indicate explicitly to participants that the interviewer was no expert in their experiences and that participants were in fact better positioned to assume the role of 'expert' in this specific domain. This reinforced the 'curious outsider' perspective that was so advantageous in the context of the EXTRA Study.

On a related note, it is vitally important that the researcher retains an inquisitive approach during the research process, showing the interviewee that they are genuinely interested in their responses without providing any indication of what would be a 'desirable' response. There are several very insightful accounts of techniques in interviewing (e.g. Breakwell & Timotijevic, 2020). However, an example or two would be beneficial. Imagine that the researcher wishes to ask the participant about their decision-making in relation to substance use or sexual behaviour. This would need to be done carefully and any terms that could potentially be misunderstood as stigmatising or pathologising the participant or their behaviour (e.g. 'substance *mis*use' or 'promiscuity') would need to be avoided. These are value-laden terms that are often used without consideration of the ripples of meaning they create. Yet, the reverse is also true—a response from the interviewer which suggests that they 'approve' of a particular behaviour could give the impression that this is what the researcher wishes to hear, which may also limit the scope of the research. The participant may be attempting to relinquish a behaviour that they do not desire which may be at odds with the interviewer's apparent endorsement of that behaviour. A robust means of addressing this is neutrality (insofar as this is possible) and to refrain from making any value judgements during the course of the interview. Close attention to the language used in interviews is of critical importance.

A key practical consideration in research is where and how the interviews will be conducted. Who will conduct the interview—the researcher or an assistant? Will the interview take place at the researcher's office or at the participant's home? Will it be voice-recorded or will notes be taken during the interview? In order to ensure that the participant is at ease, it is preferable for the interviewee to choose where the interview should be conducted, although the researcher should also be attentive to their own safety and wellbeing. An appropriate risk assessment may need to be completed as part of the ethics application. Moreover, it is of course necessary that participants provide consent for the interview to be recorded.

There can be unforeseen challenges. Some examples would be beneficial. One of the interviewees in the EXTRA Study contacted the researcher on social media and initially expressed a preference to be interviewed in her home but subsequently expressed anxieties about allowing a male interviewer into her home due to previous experiences of victimisation from men. After further discussion, the interviewee asked the researcher to proceed with the interview in her home, which went well. However, this particular case highlights the way in which previous life experiences may engender feelings of vulnerability and fear, which the interviewer does not necessarily anticipate, potentially leading to participant disengagement. In another case, a participant who agreed to be interviewed in a hired room at her local library was verbally abused by a member of the public on the way to the interview venue. She was visibly distressed when she arrived at the interview venue due to the hostility to which she had been subjected in view of her visible trans identity. Although the researcher offered to postpone the interview for another occasion, the participant was keen to proceed but was adversely affected by this experience, which resurfaced several times during the course of the interview. It was noteworthy that, in this interview, there was a focus on previous experiences of discrimination. On a similar note, another participant, who was at an early stage of her transition, asked the interviewer if she could arrive at the interview venue (a hired room in a public library) presenting as male because she was fearful of verbal abuse on the way to the interview venue. The interviewer was of course clear with the participant that she was welcome to choose how she presented during the interview. However, it was clear that the interviewee was concerned about what the interviewer would think if they were to arrive dressed in masculine clothing and that some reassurance was necessary. These issues may not be habitually considered by a researcher prior to a research study but the EXTRA Study demonstrates their relevance.

METHODOLOGICAL ASPECTS OF THE EXTRA STUDY

This section focuses on the specific methodological aspects of the EXTRA Study, namely ethics; the recruitment of participants to the study; methods of data generation and data analysis; the process of conducting the analysis and the themes that were generated. This information enables readers to understand the rationale for various methodological decisions taken during the execution of the study.

Ethical Aspects

After the study was designed, the next step was to seek ethical clearance. Ethics is a significant component of any research study which must ensure the wellbeing of both research participants and the researchers involved. Furthermore, it is vital that individuals provide *informed consent* prior to participation and that they are debriefed at the earliest opportunity. All social scientists receive ethical training and most professional associations (such as the British Psychological Society) have ethical guidelines, which must be followed by researchers and practitioners. The study was designed and conducted in accordance with British Psychological Society (2008) Code of Ethics and Conduct and was approved by the Faculty of Health and Life Sciences Ethics Committee at De Montfort University (REF: 3275). Some of the particularly noteworthy ethical considerations are described in this section.

In the context of the EXTRA Study, it was acknowledged that the project focused on several potentially sensitive issues whose ethical implications needed to be explored in the ethics application. It was acknowledged that participants may be experiencing psychological distress associated with stigmatised aspects of their identity, namely their trans gender identity and HIV status, and particularly in relation to previous experiences of stigma and prejudice. The high prevalence of poor mental health in this population was also noted. There was a risk that participation in the interview study might render salient feelings of psychological distress simply because participants might be talking about distressing experiences. However, there was no indication that participants would be *more* distressed due to the interview and, conversely, it was likely that participation in the interview might be construed as an opportunity to vocalise one's experiences and to access support if required. Indeed, all of the participants provided positive feedback to the researcher about their experience of participating in the study and many noted the 'therapeutic value' of the interview process. As discussed in Chapter 6, most participants had not disclosed their HIV status to others and reported being socially isolated, but construed the interview as an in-depth conversation with an empathic interlocutor and felt able to exchange confidences. Thus, the interview was widely described as being a therapeutic process.

When the prospective participants made contact with the researcher to express interest in being interviewed for the study, they were provided with access to the participant information sheet and asked to make contact if they decided to proceed with the interview. Individuals signed a consent form before participating—either in person or via e-mail if the participant was being interviewed over Skype. This enabled individuals to take an informed decision before participating. Only one prospective participant decided not to proceed after studying the participant information sheet. In each case, particular care was taken both to provide clarity about the aims of the project so that prospective participants knew exactly what the content of the interview would be. The researcher explicitly clarified that the participant could avoid questions that they did not wish to answer, that they could take a break during the interview if they wished to do so, and that they could withdraw from the study at any point, without giving a reason and without penalty. Crucially, participants were informed that they would still receive their £20 gift voucher even if they decided to withdraw after providing initial consent. These are of course ethical expectations of *any* research study involving human participants but these points were made exceptionally clear in the context of the EXTRA Study.

Furthermore, on the debrief sheet, participants were signposted to both local and national organisations that had expertise in supporting people with the potential stressors that participants might be facing. For instance, participants were signposted to medical, psychological and social support services in relation to their gender, HIV infection, sexual health issues and mental health. It was deemed important to provide a variety of suggestions, including online support, local support (for those who preferred to seek support in their own town or city), and national support (for those who wished to seek support outside of their own town or city, for instance because they were anxious about accessing support locally).

As noted in the subsequent chapters in Part II, participants were not generally open about their HIV status and were concerned about the potential implications of involuntary disclosure of this information to others. They were worried that this might affect their psychological well-being, relationships with others, and economic conditions. They sought assurance that their data would be completely anonymised. Participants were reassured that data from the interviews would not be traceable to them and that any information from the interviews that might increase their identifiability would be removed prior to publication. Although it is common practice to replace participants' real names with pseudonyms, this was deemed by the author to be insufficient to prevent the identification of participants. More specifically, it was thought that, given the depth of the analysis presented in this volume, use of pseudonyms might enable readers to piece together aspects of a given individual's identity and experience, potentially leading to their identification. In any case, the key aim of this volume is to shed light on the identities and experiences of trans women living with HIV in general, rather than on particular individuals. Therefore, the extracts that are presented in the remaining chapters of Part II are intended to illustrate the analytic observations, rather than to recount the story of any particular individual.

Participant Selection

In total, eleven trans women participated in the EXTRA Study. There were four criteria for eligibility: (1) self-identification as a trans woman, (2) living with HIV, (3) being at least eighteen years of age and (4) willingness to provide informed consent. All of the participants met these criteria. Thus, the focus of the study on trans women and HIV was made clear on the outset and participants were expecting to discuss intimate aspects of the lives and identities. During the course of the interview, all of the participants explicitly described themselves as trans women, although most reported identifying in other ways in the past, and wished to be referred to using the pronouns 'she/her'.

Participants were aged between thirty-one and fifty-three years. They were recruited from the following regions: London, Scotland, the West Midlands and the South East. Five participants were born in the UK and six were born abroad. Eight participants were employed and three were unemployed. One of the participants reported studying towards a university degree; eight reported GCSE/college-level qualifications; and two reported no formal education. All of the participants had been assigned male sex at birth, but self-identified as trans women. As indicated in Chapter 1, the definition of 'trans women' employed in this book is broad. It includes all individuals who were assigned male sex at birth but who now identify as trans women. It is noteworthy that the trans women who participated in this study were at distinct points in their transition journey—some had reached a point at which they were content (e.g. taking hormone replacement therapy only), while others had aspirations to continue to modify their physical appearance with surgery. All participants were undertaking hormone replacement therapy, and two participants reported having had full gender reassignment surgery and four upper surgeries only. Two participants were at a very early stage of their transition journey, having recently commenced hormone replacement therapy, and one of them self-identified as trans but focused almost exclusively on the benefits that self-presentation as female had for her ability to attract potential sexual partners, rather than their identity as a trans woman. Yet, because the individual self-identified as trans, she was deemed eligible for participation.

Participants had been living with HIV for between one and twenty-seven years and all but two of them had been diagnosed in the UK. Four participants had been diagnosed prior to their gender transition. All of the interviewees reported taking ART and all but four of them were virally suppressed. The four participants with a detectable viral load were engaged in HIV care but reported either difficulties in adhering to their HIV medication or recent diagnosis and initiation of ART. Thus, the sample was relatively heterogeneous in terms of reported experiences and identity elements that might impinge on their experience of living with HIV. For instance, it is possible that trans women diagnosed with HIV prior to their gender transition might have distinct experiences from those diagnosed after their transition. Furthermore, the stage of one's transition journey (e.g. having had full gender reassignment survey vs. having just begun the process) could also contribute to the way in which HIV is experienced. Although some qualitative research methods favour a 'relatively homogeneous sample' (Smith, Flowers, & Larkin, 2009), in this exploratory study of trans women living with HIV the diverse sample was deemed to be advantageous in order to capture a multitude of experiences.

In qualitative research studies, small sample sizes are advisable given that the focus is not on empirical generalisability but rather in-depth exploration of rich, qualitative data (Lyons & Coyle, 2007). Following other qualitative thematic analysis studies that have focused on identity and experience among sexual and gender minorities (e.g. Jaspal & Williamson, 2017), a target of ten to fifteen participants was established for the study. This was also deemed advantageous due to the exploratory nature of the study and the principal objective to generate initial, preliminary understandings of trans women's experiences of living with HIV. Given the dearth of research in the UK, it seemed important to generate

Table 4.1
Development of the
superordinate themes

Superordinate themes	Master themes
Multi-layered stigma	Anticipated and actual transphobia
	Perceived discrimination
	Fear of HIV stigma from sexual partners
Managing HIV and sex work	Economic need for sexual risk
	Positive self-presentation as a sex worker
	Sex work as an escape
Self-isolation and concealment of HIV status	Lack of social support
	Stigma and isolation
	Difficulties in HIV status disclosure
Threatened identities	Childhood trauma
	Reconciling HIV medication and hormone therapy

some overarching themes drawn from qualitative interview research in the first instance, which might subsequently inform the design of a larger research programme underpinned by different research methods in the future. Although a target of ten to fifteen participants was specified early on during the planning process, the number of participants to be included in the final sample was determined through the data saturation principle (Francis et al., 2010). After the analysis of the first seven interviews, the interview data were analysed which resulted in the superordinate themes described in this volume (see Table 4.1). Four further interviews were conducted and, given that no new themes were emerging but rather variations of the same themes were being generated, the analyses of these interviews were incorporated into these superordinate themes. They served only to enrich the existing themes, rather than to change or add to them significantly. It was evident that theoretical saturation had been achieved and, thus, further data collection ceased.

Data Collection and Analysis

The interviews were guided by a semi-structured interview schedule that tapped into self-description, self-categorisation, gender identity, sexual identity, sexual health perceptions and experiences of living with HIV. The interview schedule was constructed on the basis of previous reviews of existing research into trans people living with HIV (Jaspal, Kennedy, & Tariq, 2018; Jaspal et al., 2018). Interviews lasted between sixty and ninety minutes and were digitally recorded and transcribed verbatim. The recordings and transcripts were stored on a password-protected computer in a locked office. Interviews were conducted in participants' own preferred locations, including community centres, local libraries, participants' homes and over Skype. All participants were offered, and accepted, a £20 gift voucher and their travel expenses to the interview venue were reimbursed.

The data were analysed using an inductive, interpretative variant of thematic analysis, which has been described as 'a method which works both to reflect reality and to unpick or unravel the surface of "reality"', which provides 'a method for identifying, analyzing and reporting patterns (themes) within data' (Braun & Clarke, 2006, p. 79). It is a flexible qualitative technique that allows the analyst to identify key perceptions of, and meanings attributed to, a particular phenomenon. This approach can shed light on the subjective perceptual processes associated with participants' attempts to make sense of their experiences of living with HIV as trans women. Moreover, its idiographic mode of enquiry facilitates in-depth exploration of how each individual experiences HIV, the meanings they attribute to the condition, and how the condition is managed in the context of their trans identity. But what is a theme? A theme is essentially 'an observable pattern of meaning across a dataset which is shaped by an interrogation of what the data are telling us in relation to the original research question(s)' (Jaspal, 2020, p. 290). In the thematic analysis of the EXTRA Study, themes were derived on the basis of what the data were revealing in relation to the research questions but also in relation to the major theoretical lens that was applied to the data.

Other analytic approaches were considered, such as interpretative phenomenological analysis (Smith et al., 2009) and discourse analysis (Coyle, 2007). However, neither was considered appropriate for addressing the research questions. Interpretative phenomenological analysis has a firm commitment to phenomenology, which attempts to understand the individual's subjective experience of a given phenomenon in a 'bottom-up' manner. As outlined in Chapters 2 and 3, theories from social psychology were identified as potentially useful in adding theoretical depth to the analysis of trans women's experiences of living with HIV.

The incorporation of theory in an a priori manner appeared to challenge the fundamental principle in phenomenology of foregrounding the participant's meaning-making, which is central to interpretative phenomenological analysis. On the other hand, it was clear that the commitment of discourse analysis to social constructionism, which focuses *exclusively* on the social construction of psychological phenomena, rather than their observation, would not generate satisfactory responses to the research questions.

Epistemology

Epistemology is an important consideration for qualitative research in psychology as it determines the status of the data which are collected and the assumptions that can be made about psychological phenomena on the basis of these data. While social constructionism regards language as 'constructing, rather than reflecting, psychological and social reality', realism views language as a 'fairly accurate window into cognition, affect and experience' (Jaspal, 2020, p. 293). Some researchers view these epistemological approaches as being fundamentally at odds and, therefore, incompatible within the same research project.

Yet, complex, social psychological phenomena, such as identity, risk and psychological wellbeing, require multifaceted analyses using distinct epistemological and methodological approaches. Otherwise, it simply will not be possible to generate the depth of analysis that is required to answer the research questions that we set ourselves. For instance, in one of the interviews, a participant initially responded to the call for participants who self-identify as trans women but during the course of the interview began to self-identify as 'gender non-binary'. Through a realist lens, it would be difficult to make sense of the shift in identification within the context of a single interview because the categories 'woman' and 'gender non-binary' appear to be somewhat contradictory. However, using a social constructionist perspective, it appeared that the participant was laying claim to this identity to resist (discursively) the images, norms and values associated with dominant understandings of womanhood.

By bridging realist and social constructionist epistemological positions, it was possible to see how the *discursive* strategy of shifting between identity categories was serving an important *psychological* function of restoring feelings of coherence and compatibility. As Jaspal (2020) has argued elsewhere, we have so much to gain not only from bridging the

qualitative and quantitative paradigms but also from the various epistemological approaches espoused by researchers in psychology. Both this
example and material from the preceding chapters converge in showing
the merits of both epistemological approaches and, thus, both are incorporated in the analysis and positioned within the more flexible approach
of thematic analysis.

Doing the Analysis

Given that the analyst also conducted the interviews, he was already relatively familiar with the data. The transcripts were read repeatedly in order
for the analyst to acquire familiarity with the data. A coding scheme had
been developed in order to capture features of the transcripts that would
facilitate responses to the research questions. The coding scheme was
designed to detect aspects of the participants' accounts which captured
(1) the impact of their HIV status on the identity principles, that is, self-
esteem, continuity, self-efficacy, distinctiveness and coherence; (2) events
and situations which appear to cause psychological stress; (3) emotions,
such as guilt, anger and joy; (4) engagement in particular behaviours to
enhance the identity principles; and (5) relationships with relevant individuals and groups. It combined both realist and social constructionist
epistemological approaches.

During each reading of the transcripts, preliminary impressions and
interpretations were developed using the coding scheme. As shown in the
description of the coding scheme, these initial codes included *inter alia*
participants' meaning-making, particular forms of language, and apparent
contradictions and patterns within the data. Tenets of identity process
theory were drawn upon in order to conduct the preliminary analysis. For
instance, observations concerning the identity processes and principles
and coping strategies were made at this stage. Subsequently, these initial
codes were collated into potential themes with subsequent higher-level
interpretative work.

The analysis began after three interviews had been conducted and
seven themes were initially developed: anticipated & actual transphobia;
perceived discrimination; economic need for sexual risk; sex work as an
escape; childhood trauma positive self-presentation as a sex worker; and
stigma and isolation. An additional four interviews were conducted which
gave rise to the following additional four themes: fear of HIV stigma from
sexual partners; lack of social support; difficulties in HIV status disclosure;

and reconciling HIV medication and hormone therapy. Four more interviews were conducted and the analysis of these additional four transcripts resulted not in the generation of new themes but in the development of the existing eleven themes.

The list of eleven themes was reviewed rigorously against the qualitative data to ensure their compatibility and numerous interview extracts were listed against each corresponding theme. At this stage, specific interview extracts, which were considered representative of the themes, were selected for presentation in this volume. Finally, three of the four superordinate themes, which reflected the analysis, were developed and ordered into a coherent narrative structure. Due to space constraints, only the first three themes are discussed in this volume. See Table 4.1 for a full list of themes and superordinate themes.

DISSEMINATING THE FINDINGS

Given the dearth of data on trans women living with HIV in the UK, it was deemed essential to raise the profile of the research project but also to disseminate the emerging findings of the project to key stakeholders.

The Expert Advisory Group on Trans Health Research had been established early on in the project in order to ensure that key stakeholders, that is, researchers, community leaders, activists and the third sector workers, could contribute to the development of the research and benefit from its emerging findings. For instance, it was very important that the UK's biggest HIV charity the Terrence Higgins Trust be involved in the process because it was anticipated that the emerging findings would enable the charity to respond more effectively to the HIV prevention and care needs of trans women. Furthermore, colleagues with experience of researching other health issues in the trans population and of conducting research using different methods made very valuable contributions to the project— their constructive commentary elucidated new directions both in the EXTRA Study and in the area of HIV in trans women, more generally. Members of the trans community made fruitful contributions to the meetings, primarily because they were able to offer views on the emerging findings, assess their significance for the trans community and provide guidance on how best to engage the trans community.

During the course of the project, emerging research findings were also presented at the Trans-Forming Medicine Conference 2017: Perspectives on Transgender Healthcare. The day conference, which took place on 25 May 2017, brought together social scientists from a range of disciplines, all of whom shared an academic interest in the health and wellbeing of trans populations. The aim of presenting the emerging findings was to contextualise the issue of HIV in the broader field of trans health-care and to encourage debate about how the significant public health challenge of HIV might interact with other health issues. For instance, trans women's concerns about potential drug interactions between their hormone replacement therapy and HIV treatment; previous adverse experiences in healthcare settings; and the epidemic of poor mental health (e.g. depressive symptomatology) in trans populations were important topics of discussion. These proved to be very useful in view of the findings that emerged from the analysis.

Overview

In this chapter, key aspects of the research process were outlined in relation to the EXTRA Study. These are aspects which should be considered by researchers in relation to any qualitative study. The challenges associated with participant recruitment and establishing rapport with participants, in particular, and the possible measures that might be undertaken to address them were also described. This information is intended to be of use to other researchers who are planning to conduct research in this area. Furthermore, the specific methodological decisions taken to address the research questions were outlined. Other researchers may have taken other decisions and favoured other methodological approaches. There are of course many to choose from. It would be advantageous if the findings were 'triangulated' using other research methods. Furthermore, in this chapter, the participant sample was described in significant detail, which enables readers to understand the significance, contribution and impact of the findings presented in the remainder of the chapters in Part II.

References

Bennett, P. (1996). Dyke in academe (II). In T. A. H. McNaron & B. Zimmerman (Eds.), *The new lesbian studies: Into the twenty-first century* (pp. 3–8). New York: The Feminist Press.

Braun, V., & Clarke, V. (2006). Using thematic analysis in psychology. *Qualitative Research in Psychology, 3*(2), 77–101. https://doi.org/10.1191/147808 8706qp063oa.

Breakwell, G. M., & Timotijevic, L. (2020). Interviewing and focus groups. In G. M. Breakwell, D. B. Wright, & J. Barnett (Eds.), *Research methods in psychology* (5th ed.). London: Sage.

British Association for Sexual Health and HIV. (2019). *BASHH recommendations for integrated sexual health services for trans, including non-binary people.* http://www.gpone.wales.nhs.uk/sitesplus/documents/1000/bashh-recommendations-for-integrated-sexual-health-services-for-trans-including-non-binary-people-2019pdf.pdf.

Coloma, R. S. (2008). Border cross subjectivities and research: Through the prism of feminists of color. *Race, Ethnicity and Education, 11*(1), 11–27. https://doi.org/10.1080/13613320701845749.

Coyle, A. (2007). Discourse analysis. In E. Lyons & A. Coyle (Eds.), *Analysing qualitative data in psychology* (pp. 98–116). London: Sage.

Ellard-Gray, A., Jeffrey, N. K., Choubak, M., & Crann, S. E. (2015). Finding the hidden participant: Solutions for recruiting hidden, hard-to-reach, and vulnerable populations. *International Journal of Qualitative Methods, 14*(5), 1–10. https://doi.org/10.11772F1609406915621420.

Fay, B. (1996). *Contemporary philosophy of social science: A multicultural approach.* Cambridge: Blackwell.

Francis, J. J., Johnston, M., Robertson, C., Glidewell, L., Entwistle, V., Eccles, M. P., et al. (2010). What is an adequate sample size? Operationalising data saturation for theory-based interview studies. *Psychology & Health, 25*(10), 1229–1245. https://doi.org/10.1080/08870440903194015.

Horowitz, R. (1986). Remaining an outsider: Membership as a threat to research rapport. *Urban Life, 14,* 409–430. https://doi.org/10.11772F0098303986014004003.

Jaspal, R. (2009). 'Insider' or 'outsider'? Conducting qualitative psychological research with British South Asians. *PsyPAG Quarterly, 71,* 11–17.

Jaspal, R. (2020). Content analysis, thematic analysis and discourse analysis. In G. M. Breakwell, D. B. Wright, & J. Barnett (Eds.), *Research methods in psychology* (5th ed., pp. 285–312). London: Sage.

Jaspal, R. (in press). Stigma and HIV concealment motivation among gay men living with HIV in Finland. *Journal of Homosexuality.*

Jaspal, R., Kennedy, L., & Tariq, S. (2018). Human immunodeficiency virus and trans women: A literature review. *Transgender Health, 3*(1), 239–250. https://doi.org/10.1089/trgh.2018.0005.

Jaspal, R., Nambiar, K., Delpech, V., & Tariq, S. (2018). HIV and trans and non-binary people in the United Kingdom. *Sexually Transmitted Infections, 94*(5), 318–319. http://doi.org/10.1136/sextrans-2018-053570.

Jaspal, R., & Williamson, I. (2017). Identity management strategies among HIV-positive Colombian gay men in London. *Culture, Health and Sexuality: an*

International Journal for Research, Intervention and Care, 19(2), 1374–1388. https://doi.org/10.1080/13691058.2017.1314012.

Lyons, E., & Coyle, A. (Eds.). (2007). *Analysing qualitative data in psychology*. London: Sage. https://doi.org/10.4135/9781446207536.

Siraj, A. (2012). Looking 'in' from the 'outside': The methodological challenges of researching minority ethnic gay men and lesbian women. In S. J. Hunt & A. K. T. Yip (Eds.), *The Ashgate research companion to contemporary religion and sexuality* (pp. 59–71). Farnham: Ashgate.

Smith, J. A., Flowers, P., & Larkin, M. (2009). *Interpretative phenomenological analysis: Theory, method and research*. London: Sage.

Thompson, E. E., Neighbors, H. W., Munday, C., & Jackson, J. S. (1996). Recruitment and retention of African American patients for clinical research: An exploration of response rates in an urban psychiatric hospital. *Journal of Consulting and Clinical Psychology, 64*(5), 861–867. https://doi.org/10.1037/0022-006X.64.5.861.

CHAPTER 5

Multi-Layered Stigma

Abstract Stigma was a dominant theme in participants' accounts. The trans women who participated in the EXTRA Study described stigma due to various components of their identity, most notably their transness and HIV status. Moreover, the experience of stigma was long-standing in that individuals reported having to grapple with stigma and rejection across the life course. Most indicated that they had attempted to live their lives as gay men during adolescence and early adulthood, which had also exposed them to stigma due to homosexuality. Chronic and long-standing exposure to stigma across the life course and in various contexts, including in healthcare settings, clearly led some individuals to anticipate and fear stigma from others, which is referred to as hypervigilance. The identity principles of self-esteem and continuity were especially susceptible to threat as a result of their experiences of stigma.

Keywords Trans stigma · HIV stigma · Self-esteem · Continuity · Prejudice

EARLY REJECTION FROM SIGNIFICANT OTHERS

Interviewees reflected on early recollections, events and experiences in relation to their trans identity, focusing in particular on experiences of disclosure and their interpretation of the reactions of significant

© The Author(s) 2020
R. Jaspal, *Trans Women and HIV*,
https://doi.org/10.1007/978-3-030-57545-8_5

others, such as parents and family members. There was widespread acknowledgement of stigma which participants described as deep-rooted, long-standing and persistent since childhood:

> When I was a child of school age I was bullied and I was told I was gay because of my mannerisms which would be construed as camp rather than feminine. So being told you're gay for all of your youth makes you gay because you're told you're gay.

> They [classmates] all thought I was a freak and weird. I went to many schools.

> You could tell my parents thought I was a freak when I told them. They were speechless. Nothing to say or do because they didn't know what to say and do really. It was a traumatic time for all the family. I just thought I'll say 'I'm gay' and that opened another stressful time in my life too.

Most participants reported self-identifying as gay before acknowledging their trans identity, and many were initially exposed to homophobia. They frequently reported experiences of homophobic bullying as their feminine 'mannerisms' were pejoratively misconstrued as camp, which reportedly led them to identify publicly as gay. One participant reported internalising the stigma that she faced and attempting to live up to expectations by adopting a gay identity, rather than her true gender identity. This amounted to a strategy for protecting self-esteem, which was susceptible to threat due to pervasive social stigma. For some, coming out as gay was construed as a 'simpler' option than coming out completely as trans because they believed that being gay would at least be understood—though not necessarily approved of—by significant others. They described a context in which being trans was so poorly understood that it was almost important to articulate and share with others this significant aspect of their identity.

Moreover, participants reported developing excessive self-consciousness and feelings of insecurity due to others' responses to their transness—one interviewee was denigrated as 'a freak and weird' because of her gender non-normative behaviours and appearance, which led to a decreased sense of belonging in her school environment. She felt unable to remain in that school and changed schools repeatedly, undermining her ability to form strong friendships during childhood. Crucially, this problem persisted into adulthood and, like most interviewees, she reported feelings of loneliness as a trans adult. There was a struggle between maintaining authenticity and evading social stigma. Furthermore, it must be noted that individuals developed and, in some cases themselves acknowledged, a heightened sense of hypervigilance in that they anticipated—sometimes hastily and erroneously—stigma from others and decided to withdraw from social contexts in which this was deemed likely. Hypervigilance constituted a type of coping designed to protect identity from potential threats—specifically, to self-esteem.

This sense of hypervigilance was associated with the type of reaction that they had encountered when disclosing their trans identity to somebody that mattered to them—in particular, their parents. After all, if their parents, the most trusted significant others in their lives, did not accept them, why should anybody else? Several interviewees described their adverse experiences of confiding in their parents about their gender dysphoria, which led to psychological distress:

> It was horrible, it was horrible, I was suicidal, I tried to kill myself twice. It was hard growing up... my brothers were always on my back, my case. My dad, like at the beginning he was literally on my case about it. For them I was too neat, I was too soft, I don't wanna go play baseball, I don't wanna do masculine activities, I wanna go to the salon with my mum so it was pretty tough growing up.

> I went to a specialist boarding school and I did have a few friends but it was back when- then it was still seen as taboo, because I met another boy who was there and had the same feelings as me but he was sent away from his parents and put into this specialist boarding school with me and yeah it sort of scared me a bit...Without a thought- so I changed my name, told my parents. Their reaction's not very good so I don't talk to them anymore or my brother, but yeah, they can't accept who I am.

One interviewee felt persecuted by her brothers and father to whom she had disclosed her trans identity. This led to both suicidal ideation and two actual suicide attempts. Individuals attempted to formulate predictions about how their parents might respond to their trans identity by observing possible clues in their social context. Some described their fathers' negative appraisal of androgynous pop stars, such as Boy George, while others described the treatment of other people in their environment who had come out as gay or trans and been rejected as a result of this. Yet, in most cases, the trans women who participated in this study reported knowing of very few or no other trans people when they were growing up, which led to much uncertainty concerning others' reactions. Some believed that they would be exposed to stigma, further imperilling their sense of self-esteem. They were having to develop a 'risk assessment' (in relation to stigma and self-esteem) on the basis of little evidence.

When they did come out, some reported significant denigration due to their gender dysphoria, which led them to attempt to conceal it from others in subsequent interactions. However, for one participant, it was one of her peers whose experience shaped her approach to coming out— her peer had come out as trans and subsequently been ostracised as a result. She described this as 'scary' and noted that it discouraged her from coming out. Although the participant's parents had long suspected that she was gay, she finally disclosed her trans identity to them as an adult, which led to a breakdown in their relationship. Devoid of parental support, she felt compelled to continue her transition in the absence of this support and reported significant psychological distress when she thought about her estrangement from her family. This represented a threat to individuals' sense of continuity because the relationships that had existed were now breaking down as a result of their identity disclosure. In some cases, interviewees were given an ultimatum, that is, to 'change' or leave. Both pathways would represent a significant rupture in the psychological thread between past, present and future and were thus construed as threatening for identity.

Interviewees reported childhood experiences of stigma and rejection by significant others due to their gender non-normative behaviour, which was interpreted by others as evidence of homosexuality, rather than their transness. As demonstrated below, some reported rejecting prototypically 'masculine' behaviours and traits, in favour of 'feminine' behaviours and traits and, thus, being rejected by their siblings and parents. The psychological trauma induced by such experiences was clearly evident in participants' accounts—some experienced suicidal ideation:

And I said to him [her father] I feel like I'm a girl, and he said well you're not a girl, and then he said to me straight up, I'm not raising any gay under my roof so figure it out, and it was tough. I always ask my dad why he told me that.

Not being understood, being mislabelled and just put down, it all led me to think about ending my life.

Individuals reported that their significant others had been unable to understand what they were trying to communicate to them, namely, that they identified as female, and misconstrued them as 'gay'—an identity which was also stigmatised. The perception that one's identity was misunderstood by significant others was widespread in the participant sample. As exhibited above, parents sometimes assumed that their son was gay and subjected them to homophobic victimisation. Many had hoped that their significant others would respond more favourably, understanding and accepting their identity, and experienced a rupture in their present experiences and hopes for the future. This was challenging for their sense of continuity.

Some interviewees reported confiding in friends about their trans identity in order to derive support. However, many also described situations of rejection from these trusted others:

> Well I have some gay friends and they feel that the trans situation may not be right for me, so there's that as well with my friends where they don't necessarily feel that it's right for me because I've been I think it's mainly because I've been in a gay background and they sort of know me, they've always known me as a gay man.... I have a friend called [names friend] which is, he's another guy, he's a gay guy. Our relationship... [we] have always been quite good friends. But really as gay men. So he was out as a gay friend when I needed the HIV services and he was quite happy to be friends with me. But obviously not so supportive with me with the trans situation.

Several interviewees reported having established a circle of mainly gay friends who accepted them as gay men but provided support with this (inauthentic) identity. Most interviewees did initially attempt to construct a gay identity—some of them misattributed their gender dysphoria to homosexuality, while others initially presented themselves as gay in order to derive social acceptance (i.e. because being gay was deemed to be more socially acceptable than being trans). When they subsequently came out as trans, some individuals encountered negative reactions from their gay friends who did not 'feel that it's right for me' and who had 'always known me as a gay man'. On the one hand, gay friends did not seem to understand their trans identity and, on the other hand, they appeared to construe their coming out as trans as a 'rupture' of *their* sense of continuity. They apparently could not assimilate and accommodate the change that this represented to their friendship and, thus, rejected their friends. Yet, the inability of significant others to accept them undermined participants' ability to construct an identity characterised by authenticity.

Indeed, several interviewees described specific friends who had provided support but subsequently stigmatised or rejected them when they came out as trans:

> My best mate who was really my rock growing up just said that she couldn't just stand by and watch me mutilate myself and it was obvious she saw me as an embarrassment so stopped taking my calls, answering my calls, stopped seeing me and we just dripped apart. I was pretty devastated about that.

In the face of widespread stigma and rejection from family members, individuals commonly turned to a trusted friend with the hope and expectation that they would continue to derive social support from them. While the participant (above) had been supported by her (female) best friend when she initially came out as a gay man, describing her as 'my rock', she felt rejected by her trusted friend when she subsequently revealed that she was in fact trans. Like several interviewees, she reported not only rejection but also denigration of her trans identity since her best friend also described transitioning as 'self-mutilation' and construed it as 'an embarrassment'. It is easy to see how stigma from significant others, such as family members and trusted friends who were initially supportive, may serve to crystallise the feelings of stigma surrounding trans identity and potentially lead to self-stigma. These early experiences of rejection were aversive for both the continuity and self-esteem principles of identity.

BEING TRANS: A STIGMATISED IDENTITY

In addition to these early experiences of stigma and rejection, all of the participants reported experiencing stigma in adulthood as they began to crystallise and share with others their trans identity. Having taken the initial decision to disclose their trans identity to significant others, they began to share it on a wider scale, which resulted in a range of reactions. Stigma was anticipated and experienced in a multitude of contexts. In particular, individuals reported stigma from cisgender gay men:

> Gay men aren't particularly nice to trans women, especially ones that identified as gay men before. So my mass exodus of friends wasn't when I was

diagnosed as positive. It was when I came out as trans so that's not the problem, not the HIV part, the T-part being not really that welcomed and trans people don't feel that welcomed in the lesbian gay community generally and that's a problem.

I experienced that [stigma] in Soho because I went to a coffee bar one time and I went as trans and I had had a horrible response from gay men, which I was upset about because if they saw me in a different light as they saw me on the gay side they mostly would have been very different towards me so I know that there is a lot of stigma from gay men and on the gay scene in general towards trans women.

There is a lot of stigma from gay men and on the gay scene in general towards trans women.

There's a lot of misogyny in the gay community. There's a lot of men that are virgins that never had any intimacy with a woman, that are complete vagina phobic, that are really quite nasty and while that's so prevalent in the LGBT community, trans people are marginalised even further and pushed away into their own smaller group and therefore not accepted to make things even harder to be HIV-positive and trans.

Participants unanimously challenged the notion that the 'LGBT community' is cohesive and unified and emphatically noted the stigma directed at them by gay men, in particular. Several described the dismay that gay men expressed in response to 'coming out' as trans, especially when the trans person had formerly identified as gay. This suggested that there was a perception of 'treachery' in that, in disclosing her trans identity, a trans woman was perceived to be relinquishing her gay identity. Similarly, as observed above, participants described their attempts to derive social support from the gay friends who rejected them. This undermined individuals' sense of belonging in a context in which they hoped to be accepted. In fact, individuals expected to be accepted because of the perception that sexual and gender minorities share a common sense of being a minority in a heteronormative and cisgenderist world and were disappointed to observe that their transness was also subject to social stigma from trusted others. The early experience of rejection, which undermined self-esteem, persisted in adulthood.

Some interpreted gay men's rejection of trans women as a form of misogyny, thereby demonstrating the depth and severity of perceived transphobia from gay men. Crucially, they also noted that lesbian women were dismissive of trans women because of their belief that trans women are not 'real' women. This exhibits a pervasive threat to belonging among trans women in lesbian, gay and bisexual circles. This thwarted sense of belonging in lesbian, gay and bisexual circles—and the loneliness it entails—was identified as aggravating the psychological burden of living with HIV. Rejection from gay men and lesbian women must be considered a multi-faceted threat to belonging, since there was also a pervasive sense of general marginalisation:

> I'm laughed at every day in the street and called 'tranny' and all these other slurs.

> I know there's some people look at me and think 'oh, that's some sort of trans person, tranny-type person' and other people look at me and sort of take a second look.

Understandably, repeated experiences of stigma, denigration and rejection led interviewees to experience low self-esteem and negative emotions and to employ strategies for coping with the threats induced by such experiences. Some participants reportedly wished to expedite their full gender transition in order to avoid denigrating remarks from others:

> Because I'm scared, I'm really scared and shy of-of just- of yeah of rejection, maybe? I'm just really, really scared, I just know that I want to change facially before I can do it.

> I dress like this because it's- I'm trying to please society and- and- and one thing- because...I'm really afraid of rejection and I'm really afraid of being bullied or called names.. When I dress, I do it privately. I try not to go in public.

As noted above, one participant opted to present as male in contexts in which she perceived a high risk of stigma, which led to decreased feelings of identity authenticity. Her account captured her desire to conform to societal expectations by presenting as male in contexts in which denigration, bullying and rejection were perceived to be likely. Some interviewees opted for self-presentation in ways perceived to be socially acceptable to the detriment of identity authenticity because of the significant psychological burden of stigma. Indeed, given long-standing exposure to stigma, many found this to be deeply distressing and, thus, took measures to avoid it.

Similarly, others reported leading a 'double life' in relation to their transness, expressing their trans identity in 'safe' contexts and concealing it in those construed as risky:

> I was still living a bit of a double life...dressing in a feminine way but gender neutral but mm what you would say feminine but also a bit boyish so yeah. It was last year that I decided that I can't keep on doing this. It's depressing. It's driving me nuts.

> I just lived life as a male and just did normal things and it was just getting to me... I just got a bit fed up a bit in the end, it's not really me and that's not what I want.

> I just tried being a man. I just tried to live, to be a father and I just couldn't.

Passing is a coping strategy whereby the individual feigns membership of a group of which they are not really a member (Breakwell, 1986). The strategy of passing ('trying to be a man' and 'doing normal things') was pervasively employed to reduce the risk of identity threat and to satisfy others' expectations. The strategy—though fruitful in the short term—was rejected after a period of time given that it too caused distress. A lack of authenticity can cause threats to identity and the strategy of passing is associated with feelings of anxiety about involuntary disclosure of the concealed identity element. The fear of being 'found out' was psychologically challenging for some interviewees who believed that they would be rejected, as they had been early on in their lives, if their 'secret' were revealed.

Similarly, one participant who attended her interview dressed as a male explained this decision by noting that she was 'trying to please society', on the one hand, and that she feared rejection from others, on the other hand. Her coping strategy focused on decreasing the risk of stigmatising remarks that might undermine self-esteem or belonging. However, her sense of authenticity was clearly compromised by the strategy of passing given her complete disidentification with her male presentation. Crucially, there was considerable fear about the consequences of attempting to find a balance between authentic self-presentation (as a woman) and inauthentic passing (as a man) in order to avoid social stigma. They were acutely aware of the need to demonstrate to others, including health-care professionals, their commitment to the gender into which they were transitioning in order to gain acceptance as women (Pearce, 2018). This balancing act thus represented a significant psychological dilemma—their accounts highlighted the threat to psychological coherence since they found it challenging to reconcile a socially acceptable public identity with their authentic gender identity.

In addition to the pervasive denigration of trans women, 'fetishisa-tion' was also noted as a form of stigma which caused some trans women distress:

> And so a lot of people that want to shag somebody that's trans it is a fetishistic sort of thing rather than a meeting of minds [laughs] so I thought I can't deal with that and being public with it as well I can't change either of those things so it was kind of enforced celibacy I suppose which yeah it was hard I guess but, as I say at that time it was really messy because of the other people involved so I didn't really have the energy for any of that sort of thing.

It was widely recognised that some cisgender men have a sexual prefer-ence for trans women, which was construed as a purely sexual, rather than romantic or emotional, preference. Participants referred to the prolifera-tion of pornography featuring trans women and lamented the terms that were frequently used to describe them (e.g. 'trannies' and 'chicks with dicks'). Several construed this as a form of stigma partly because they did not feel that their feminine identity was validated by men but rather that their transness was being fetishised. Most interviewees lamented the focus on sexual behaviour and some opted for 'enforced celibacy', that is, the avoidance of any sexual relations, because they doubted the emotional depth of their relationships with men. In some cases, they believed that they were being fetishised due to their transness. While some found this acceptable, others rejected this as a form of objectification by men and resisted relationships. This avoidance strategy was designed to limit expo-sure to fetishisation, which they construed as a form of stigma. Yet, it also deprived them of potential sources of social support and increased feel-ings of loneliness and isolation. Many did wish to find a partner but one who valued them as people, not just because they were trans women.

In view of pervasive stigma, several participants internalised trans-phobic stigma and appeared to accept its veracity but sought to distance themselves from stigmatising traits which they perceived to be attributed to trans women:

> For me I wake up in the morning and the first thing I think about is what I would like to do today to be a better me than yesterday? Whereas [other trans women think] 'today I'll wake up and be like okay where am I gonna get my next weed from?' Or, 'where am I gonna get my next sniff from? Or, when am I gonna get my boob job?' Or, 'I wanna have smaller hips y'know?' And then there's the rush, there's the 'go and get pumped, go and get pills, self-medicate', so it does a lot of negative- that go on in the trans world.

> But I think it's really terrible that people look down on us, or even when I first got diagnosed with HIV, I was hammered about if I was an escort and I'm like no, this is a situation where I am in a relationship for 5 years and he's the one cheating outside and brought it home to me. That's how I ended up getting diagnosed. It was not a situation of me being an escort.

Some interviewees appeared to accept and express negative social stereotypes of trans women—as superficial, involved in sex work, addicted to drugs. Crucially, they constructed and manifested a distinctive identity which clearly differentiated them from these negative stereotypes. They stigmatised other trans women and presented themselves as different from *them*. There was an emerging 'us versus them' dynamic in their self-construal as 'good' trans women versus stereotypically 'bad' trans women. A source of threat for some participants was the assumption that people reportedly made concerning the source of their HIV infection—namely whether one had been an escort, alluding to the high prevalence of sex work among trans women. As demonstrated above, the participant attributed sex work to *other* trans women, distancing it from her own identity. In short, there was an attempt to deflect stigma (and to protect self-esteem) by disassociating oneself from negative stereotypes of trans women.

Stigma in Healthcare

It has been observed that trans women report high levels of stigma in healthcare settings, which can lead to disengagement and decreased help-seeking. In addition to having actual experiences of stigma in healthcare settings, they may anticipate stigma due to pervasive experiences of stigma in other contexts. The trans women who participated in this study described different forms of stigma experienced in healthcare settings:

> So for me now being trans, first off in the hospital it was drama, because obviously they put me on the women's ward because obviously they know I was trans, speaking to people and having a bit of privacy was difficult, because obviously everyone is there in the open. It was- it was very uncomfortable, it- it was not a comfortable sit- I mean you're already going through a trauma or situation where you wanna seek medical help but yet you don't have that comfort, does that make sense?

> I've been put in all kinds of difficult situations because of my health needs, like in the NHS and it's not always intentional but it's like a kind of stigma situation because they don't get my life, who I am, or my needs. Do they want to know? I don't know. Are they just closing their eyes to us? I don't know.

There was a pervasive perception among participants that decreased understanding of trans identity and healthcare needs reflected a type of stigma. First, it was often stated that healthcare practitioners did not acquire training in relation to trans people because of a perception that trans people's healthcare needs are of lesser importance than those of cisgender people. They expected to be understood and felt helpless when healthcare practitioners seemed, or reported being, unable to provide effective healthcare. Participants doubted that their needs were incorporated into medical training and attributed this absence of knowledge to the invisibility of trans people in the context of healthcare. The perception that they were not been treated effectively was challenging for self-efficacy since they perceived no control over their situation or the care that they received. Second, some interviewees believed that decreased understanding of trans identity and needs could be attributed to an intentional ignorance, that is, the desire not to know or learn. As noted above, participants reported feeling uncomfortable in healthcare settings because of the decreased understanding of their needs as trans women. One respondent proceeded to describe how decreased understanding of the healthcare needs impacted her:

> But she [her HIV doctor] just didn't understand the transgender part of it [her healthcare] and that's when she ended up sending me to Dean Street 'cause she's like they would have more of an understanding, 'cause I was

y'know explaining about my hormones and how at the time, I was taking like eight pills a day, plus my hormone pills, that would be twelve- sixteen pills a day in total, so it's kind of like asking her if patches would work better and then I don't have to take the hormone pills I can only focus on taking my HIV pills and she's like she can't- she don't know, she don't have knowledge of it so I had to end up now stop hormones completely focus on my HIV medications only, so I just totally- so my whole transition just went a bit backwards, growing hair again and stuff, so that was pretty difficult.

Several interviewees described the psychologically adverse experience of being treated by an HIV physician who did not understand their broader healthcare needs. The focus of the above participant's treatment was reportedly her HIV infection, which, though important, did not fully address her total healthcare needs, as a trans woman. She was compelled to cease hormone replacement therapy in order to address her HIV infection, which negatively affected her transition and, thus, her identity. Although the focus was on treating a serious health condition, namely HIV, which was viewed by doctors as a clinical priority, HIV was not always the sole clinical priority for the trans women who participated in this study:

When I was diagnosed, yes, it was scary but my first thought was 'what does this mean for my hormones and my transition?' I said it to my doctor and he was just like 'we've got bigger issue to deal with'. I mean, who does he think he is? I'd rather be dead as a woman, than alive with a penis.

Some interviewees noted that their transition was viewed by doctors as less important than their HIV infection, which was construed as stigmatising. This reinforced the view that their trans identity was not taken seriously, that it was poorly understood, and that its significance for them as trans women was underestimated by healthcare practitioners. This led some patients to express anxiety about continuing to engage with HIV care and, in some cases, to disengage from it. As the extract above indicated, individuals were generally cognisant of the potential consequences of disengaging from HIV care but were willing to do so in order to proceed with their transition in an uninterrupted manner. They were willing to take the risk if it meant that they were able to continue with the transition. In short, their transition was the clinical priority for them but this was not perceived to be the view of healthcare practitioners who appeared to prioritise their HIV treatment. This essentially reflected a strategy for maintaining a sense of continuity, since individuals had embarked upon their transition journey in order to create consistency in identity. By discontinuing their hormone replacement therapy, they ran the risk of identity *dis*continuity.

Crucially, there is no evidence that HIV treatment and hormone replacement therapy are necessarily incompatible (Radix, Sevelius, & Deutsch, 2016). However, this is not always understood by trans women and, as suggested in the accounts above, by physicians and other health-care practitioners. Effective physician-patient communication is vital. In the interviewee's case, she felt stigmatised because HIV treatment was presented as the 'bigger issue'. As noted above, it is important to note that the experience of having to disengage from hormone replacement therapy was perceived as a significant setback in their transition journey and some reported experiencing negative memories of their 'former self' which in turn represented previous identity threat:

> Stopping the hormones was like being my former self again, basically a boy on the outside. I wanted to die because I was getting hair back and it was like hitting rewind.

As exemplified by this account, the process of interrupting hormone replacement therapy represented a significant threat to the continuity principle of identity since the past ('my former self') was being rendered salient. The present and future seemed regressive and uncertain.

In addition to perceived implicit stigma, interviewees described overt stigma in healthcare settings associated with both their trans identity and HIV status:

> A dentist has not wanted to do my teeth [because of her HIV status] to the point that they were rotting completely out and I had to go to the hospital- taken to hospital and have them done, then again I don't tell a lot of people my positive situation because of the stigma and that so.

> I was there for my bloods and you could just see it in his eyes and what he was thinking. He was thinking I must be a prostitute. I even think I heard him whispering that to a nurse but I can't be sure of it.

> The only time I had a negative experience from a health or- was when I had my reviews for my disability money, when I said I was HIV-positive

and doing like an exam on my body he would go and wash his hands or ah- he asked me to- go and wash his hands constantly and it put me off, a bit of oh, is he washing his hands because he thinks he can get it from touching me or what?

Several interviewees reported being excluded from healthcare settings due to their HIV-positive status. Some reported being refused dental-care. Indeed, stigma in this particular healthcare setting was pervasive. Some interviewees reported that, when they disclosed their HIV status to their dentist, they were frequently given appointments at the end of the day. Some dentists indicated to them that this was a measure to decrease the risk of HIV transmission to other patients, while others provided no explanation. The observation that healthcare practitioners were washing their hands more frequently than they might ordinarily do when treating other patients was construed as stigmatising. Often, interviewees attributed this to their HIV status and to the perception (among healthcare practitioners) that they might contract HIV through touching. Similarly, as noted above, individuals suspected that health-care practitioners made assumptions about their involvement in sex work when they disclosed their HIV status, with one participant reporting that they thought that she had heard the doctor say this to a nurse explicitly. Another participant that her bladder examination was postponed until the end of the day so that the room could be 'sterilised' given that she was living with HIV:

> I had to go for a bladder examination about two years ago... And they came back and this is about lunch time, and then they came back and said oh, we're not gonna do the- the bladder examination thing until the end of the day, because we have to sterilise the room after you've been in... so there's little things like that, that obviously still come up.

> When doctors, experts are telling you you're diseased and contagious, sometimes it gets to you a bit and you started thinking that they know what they're talking about so it must be true.

These experiences crystallised the perception of stigma in interviewees' minds, leading some to rethink the benefits of disclosing their HIV status to healthcare practitioners. Some began to internalise the stigma that they encountered, especially as it was directed at them by 'experts'. It accentuated the already heightened state of hypervigilance in relation to what others were saying and thinking about trans people, leading some to believe that stigma was perhaps more pervasive than it actually was. As noted in Chapter 6, stigmatising experiences of this kind contributed to non-disclosure of one's HIV status and to increased self-isolation behaviours.

COPING WITH HIV STIGMA

In addition to the various other forms of stigma, HIV stigma surfaced as a pervasive theme in participants' accounts. All of the interviewees described HIV as a stigmatising trait and, although one of them reported having come to terms with her HIV status, they consensually feared stigma on the basis of their positive serostatus:

> When I found out, I just felt really shocked and dirty and actually the first thought was 'how long I got now?'

> I was really worrying about what other people was gonna say about me being positive, HIV, I mean...They'd definitely know I was prostituting myself.

> The problem is if somebody find out [about being HIV-positive], everybody gonna start talking and then you gonna be in a bad image...they make you feel bad.

Participants' reported reactions to testing positive for HIV were similar to those reported in other populations. They drew on negative characteristics and social representations, which are commonly associated with HIV, such as being 'dirty', immortality and sexual promiscuity. They expressed concern that these negative characteristics would be applied to them and they would be stigmatised as a result. There was also some evidence of internalised HIV stigma, whereby individuals themselves uncritically accepted the stigmatising social representations of HIV that they acknowledged. Since they themselves accepted these representations, it seemed foreseeable that others, to whom they disclosed their HIV status, would do the same. As indicated earlier, there was a sense of hypervigilance in the participant sample and they feared that they would become the subject of gossip. They felt nervous about disclosing their HIV status which amounted to a strategy for protecting self-esteem.

All of the participants reported actual past experiences of stigma and rejection due to their HIV status. They alluded to the threat to self-esteem associated with HIV stigma, which led many to conceal her HIV status. Some actively denied HIV stigma in order to cope with it:

> I do get a lot of stigma because I get a sense that I've like got to tell a guy I'm going with but I just shut my mind to it really, just take it through one ear and out the other because it's easy than just like over-thinking it.

> Sometimes I just tell myself 'no, I've not been stigmatised' even though yes it is bloody obvious that I have.

> I push those experiences [of HIV stigma] to the back of my mind basically.

In view of the potential threats to self-esteem associated with exposure to HIV stigma, some interviewees reported attempting to suppress thoughts about their previous experiences of such stigma. This was deemed preferable to 'over-thinking' their experiences of stigma. There were also reports of some re-thinking the nature of their experience, with some reporting that the experience that they had had may not be 'stigma'. By denying the true nature and meaning of the experience, they were more able to avoid the negative implications for the self-esteem principle of identity. Such experiences led several individuals to construe HIV stigma as pervasive and to conceal their HIV status from others.

Interviewees discussed their feelings when they were confronted with HIV stigma, which suggested psychological distress:

> I remember being rejected at the last minute by this one guy I liked. I remember going down in the lift [of his apartment] and just crying all the way.... It was just that feeling of being dirty or just repulsive to him.

> You never do get used to the stigma side. Each blow hurts as much as the last.

These extracts highlighted the significant threats to self-esteem associated with HIV stigma. Participants described their own internalisation of the stigma that they encountered, uncritically accepting the notion that they were 'dirty' or 'repulsive' because of their HIV status. Although individuals had developed strategies for attempting to cope with HIV stigma, such as denial, reconceptualisation of the experience and non-disclosure, some noted that it was impossible to adapt to HIV stigma and that each experience was aversive for identity. Another participant elaborated her experience of being diagnosed with HIV in view of her other stigmatised identity elements:

> To be honest, I found the whole HIV thing a bit overwhelming, you know, because I've barely got through one hoop and then the second, third and now there's this one. It's like, what do I have going for me, if anything?

This extract illustrates the challenge faced by most interviewees who reported that they had barely come to terms with the stigma associated with their perceived homosexuality and trans identity, which rendered the experience of being diagnosed with HIV 'overwhelming' for identity. More specifically, some felt devoid of any social or psychological resources to cope with the stigma of HIV given that they already felt unable to cope with stigma due to their other identity elements. The threat to self-esteem was evident, as some began to doubt their self-worth due to their HIV diagnosis.

Consistent with the observation that individuals developed hyper-vigilance in response to the stigma that they had experienced, several interviewees anticipated that reactions from potential sexual partners would be negative and that it would therefore be difficult to disclose their HIV status to them:

> The HIV side can be quite difficult sometimes, obviously if you explain it to someone you've got HIV....I do, I do think about it sometimes. Because I'm trying to work out the [...] as a trans female how I would go about telling men that I'm HIV positive. Whatever happens whether you get stigma when you tell men or yes I don't know.... My thought was I told people they wouldn't go with me. That they would automatically reject me because I was HIV.

> Well that fear comes from sort of like rejection, being rejected because I know that in [my] world I would most likely be going with heterosexual guys so it's... I'm not quite sure how I would tell them.

> Yeah it depends on the person really I've a couple of friends who still can't really get their heads round it and they mention it quite a lot, so I've tried to distance myself from them I guess.

Some participants were especially concerned about HIV stigma as a result of the change in their sexual contacts. For instance, having presented as gay men previously, some interviewees were concerned about how heterosexual men (with whom they anticipated having sex) would react to their HIV status. They noted decreased knowledge of HIV among heterosexual men which might lead to rejection. One strategy was to limit the risk of such a situation by distancing themselves from individuals who might stigmatise them due to their HIV status.

OVERVIEW

In this chapter, the multiple layers of stigma experienced by trans women living with HIV have been described. These experiences of stigma are long-standing in that they stem from childhood and persist in adulthood. Stigma is faced in various contexts—at home, from sexual partners and in healthcare settings. Due to these adverse experiences of stigma, trans women living with HIV in the UK may experience threats to multiple principles of identity—especially to self-esteem and continuity. They may strive to construct positive distinctiveness from 'other' trans women. Moreover, chronic exposure to stigma can lead some to develop a sense of hypervigilance, whereby trans women living with HIV anticipate stigma and attribute potentially innocuous events and situations to stigma. This in turn can lead some to opt for identity concealment and self-isolation, rather than identity disclosure and the derivation of social support. This is discussed further in the next chapter.

REFERENCES

Breakwell, G. M. (1986). *Coping with threatened identities*. London: Methuen.

Pearce, R. (2018). *Understanding trans health: Discourse, power and possibility*. Bristol: Policy Press.

Radix, A., Sevelius, J., & Deutsch, M. B. (2016). Transgender women, hormonal therapy and HIV treatment: A comprehensive review of the literature and recommendations for best practices. *Journal of the International AIDS Society, 19*(3, Suppl. 2), 20810. https://doi.org/10.7448/IAS.19.3.20810.

CHAPTER 6

Self-Isolation and Identity Concealment

Abstract In response to threats to identity associated with social stigma, trans women living with HIV in the UK may resort to identity concealment and self-isolation. In some contexts, they conceal their trans identity by presenting as male and, in others, they may attempt to pass as female (in a binary sense). The concealment of one's HIV status—especially from sexual partners—was a prevalent strategy for protecting identity from threat due to previous experiences of hostility in the context of HIV status disclosure. The perceived social and economic costs of HIV status disclosure are described. These can inhibit HIV status disclosure, which in turn can impede the derivation of social support in the face of an HIV diagnosis. Trans women living with HIV may become reliant on individualised, less effective strategies for coping.

Keywords Self-isolation · Identity concealment · Authenticity · Belonging · Social support

CONCEALING TRANS IDENTITY

Most participants described difficulties in relation to disclosing various aspects of their identity. All of the participants reported being judged and stigmatised by significant others during childhood and in later adulthood when they attempted to come out as trans. As outlined in previous

© The Author(s) 2020   109
R. Jaspal, *Trans Women and HIV*,
https://doi.org/10.1007/978-3-030-57545-8_6

chapters, exposure to stigma due to this fundamental component of identity can be threatening. A key strategy for attempting to cope with threat and for limiting exposure to social stigma was to conceal one's trans identity from others. For instance, one participant was sceptical about disclosing her trans identity to others at university, although she was considering it:

> I'm considering coming out [as trans and as being HIV-positive] to my university because they do have a disability department and they're quite friendly- they take their confidentiality very seriously, yes, at the end I know it is not like this- not in the UK but- I was afraid when I was- when I was making my applications I was afraid that if I write down that I'm transsexual I'm not gonna get elected, and I want to get elected and at the same time, yes I'm afraid that you know, if I come out as transsexual then people in my industry are going to know subsequently or yes, occasionally I think people- people that I don't want to know who will be targeting me and there'll be gossip, yes and that is never a positive one, people are very judgmental.

Some individuals may not seek, or be able to access, support services because of the anticipated consequences of doing so. They were essentially deprived of possible support and, thus, had to rely on other less effective coping strategies. The participant (above) was concerned that she might not even be admitted to university, as a trans person living with HIV, and thus refrained from disclosing this information to others. Similarly, several interviewees expressed fear in relation to 'gossip' and 'judgmental' responses from others. There was a clear sense of vulnerability due to both the trans and HIV-positive elements of their identity, given the possible stigma and rejection that might ensue from their involuntary disclosure. It is also important to note that some of the interviewees were unaware of legislation in the UK protecting them from discrimination due to protected characteristics, including their gender. They believed that discrimination on the basis of their trans identity was possible, largely because it was commonplace in their countries of origin, and that they would receive no institutional support in the UK to counteract it. Indeed, in other studies it has been shown that migrants to the UK may base their risk appraisal (in relation to stigma and protection) on their experiences of stigma and institutional support in their home countries (e.g. Jaspal, 2014).

For some participants and particularly those at an earlier stage of their transition, they attempted to cope by presenting as male in contexts in which social stigma was anticipated:

> I dress like this [as male] because it's- I'm trying to please society and one thing- because I told you at the beginning I'm really afraid of rejection and I'm really afraid of being bullied or called names I don't want my transition to be- to transition, in other words, I don't wanna go- when I dress, I do it privately.

Although the participant identified as a trans woman, she did report presenting as male in most contexts because she did not believe that she passed as a woman and believed that being identifiable as a trans woman would expose her to social stigma. Actual and anticipated experiences of bullying evoked memories of identity threat due to her gender and sexuality during childhood (see Chapter 5), which in turn reinforced these feelings in adulthood. In order to avoid this, she presented as male, which also had implications for her sense of identity authenticity since she did not view her self-presentation as congruent with her actual identity. There was a discernible tension between the social and psychological levels of identity, therefore. Yet, the concealment of her trans identity in contexts in which social stigma was deemed likely was the preferable strategy for protecting identity.

Similarly, participants who were born outside the UK described their experience of leaving their native countries and distancing themselves from significant others, namely their parents, family members and close friends, whom they loved but among whom they could not 'be my true self':

> They [British people] always say we [migrants] come here for economic situations but actually no for me it was to escape the bullying and judgement. Only here I can be a trans woman, not in my country an if I go back I will go back to wearing trousers with short hair to hide it, because I can't be myself, not my true self.

The participant (above) also self-identified as a trans woman but reported shifting between masculine and feminine self-presentation in order to conceal her trans identity from significant others who, she believed, did not and would not accept her trans identity. As outlined in Chapter 5, this coping strategy was partly effective for protecting her from social stigma but was severely threatening for her sense of identity authenticity since she was compelled to 'play a role' which was inconsistent with her intrapsychic self-construal. The few participants who adopted this coping strategy also reported fear in relation to involuntary disclosure of their trans identity to individuals from whom they sought to conceal it. They described the challenges in maintaining and 'protecting' their projected masculine identity to these groups and individuals, including their attempts to ensure that there was little or no communication between groups or individuals who may 'share' this information against their will:

> When I go to my country, my friends say 'ah bring your friend next time' and here they [my friends] want to know about my country but in my country I have no English friends and here I have no family. It's hard for me.

This reflected engagement in both the 'passing' and compartmentalisation strategies for protecting identity. On the one hand, individuals attempted to 'pass' as masculine or feminine in relevant social contexts and, on the other hand, they attempted to compartmentalise their identities in accordance with social context so that only the 'congruent' self-presentation was enacted in each context. This was psychologically taxing for trans women in this position because there remained a risk of involuntary disclosure of the identity that they strove to conceal. Yet, for other participants, this strategy was utilised even in intragroup contexts, that is, in LGBT contexts, in which they had hoped to derive social support.

Due to the pervasive stigma that they faced in LGBT settings, several respondents felt uneasy about frequenting LGBT spaces. They had experienced, and anticipated further, discrimination and therefore decided to disengage from these settings. This essentially deprived them of any possible social support from other sexual and gender minority individuals in these settings, as noted in the following extracts:

> So, I'm not the typical transgender gay person at all really, I do mingle with certain aspects of the LGB community and then on the other side I don't really want much to do with them because I find their- a lot of them are hypocritical, there are a lot of hypocritical people in the LGB community so.

> I just get a lot of looks when I go out on the gay scene because there's a lot of transphobia about so I don't go much. I just keep myself to myself.

Interviewees reported anticipating social support in LGBT settings because of the shared minority identity of most people who frequent these spaces but encountered hostile attitudes and 'hypocritical people'. There was a sense that they could not rely on other people in these contexts which essentially closed all possible avenues of social support. Trans women who experience and anticipate stigma in LGBT settings may find it difficult to discuss aspects of their trans identity with other people. They may come to believe that people do not understand their identity and that they are unwilling to accept it. Consequently, there is a risk that they may come to rely on individualised and less effective coping strategies, such as self-isolation and identity concealment, as a means of protecting identity from threat.

Given that several interviewees also reported self-stigma in relation to various elements of their identity, including their transness, there is also a risk that this self-stigma is perpetuated and that there is no social recourse from it (i.e. through the derivation of social support). After all, self-disclosure and exchanging confidences are known to be effective strategies for responding to stigma since individuals are empowered to develop alternative ways of thinking through exposure to more positive social representations of their identity (Breakwell, 1986). In view of the stifling stigma that many experienced, it is concerning that few of the participants in this study felt able to derive social support from other LGBT people.

As noted in Chapter 5, participants were also aware of another form of stigma, namely the 'fetishisation' of trans women—both in LGBT spaces and among heterosexual men—which led them to disengage from these contexts:

> I don't want to be some guy's play thing, as a trans woman, so I just don't tell them unless necessary, you know.

While some individuals were receptive to the sexual attention that they received from others (as trans women), many also noted that they wished to form non-sexual relationships—both platonic and romantic. They construed the 'fetishisation' of trans women as a barrier to the formation and maintenance of such relationships and, thus, disengaged from contexts in which they believed that they would be fetishised. This too amounted to a form of self-imposed self-isolation and identity concealment. In short, there was a view that they would not derive the type of relationship (or support) that they required, rendering engagement in these settings futile for their identity needs.

Interviewees who were early on in their transition journey (i.e. those who wished to undergo gender reassignment surgery but who had not yet done so) expressed trepidation about presenting as female in some contexts because they believed that they would face rejection due to their inability to pass as female:

> I prefer to change properly before being open about trans.

The participant (above) preferred to wait until she had undergone further hormone replacement therapy and gender reassignment surgery before presenting as female in all contexts because she feared stigma and rejection from others. She was fearful of others' responses to her identity as a trans woman and, thus, wished to pass completely as female because presenting in a way that was consistent with her psychological sense of gender identity. Crucially, she did not believe that she would be accepted as a trans woman and therefore sought to pursue, construct and present to others a binary female identity, rather than a trans identity. At several points during the interview, the interviewee described her desire to 'erase' her previous male identity because of its associations with negative and traumatic aspects of her past:

> I want to just forget it all, everything before that because it's an unhappy time for me, my life, and I want to just be a woman because that's how I'm happy.

It was clear that the desire to erase her past was attributable to the negative experiences that she had faced while presenting as male, that is, the stigma and denigration that she had experienced. This included homophobia, since she presented as a gay man, but also rejection from men whom she found desirable. She reported being attracted to 'manly men' who identified as heterosexual and noted that only a binary female self-presentation would render her attractive to those whom she desired. This in turn led her to pursue a binary identity which reportedly would pave the way to a happier and more fulfilling life. Due to pervasive stigma, a trans identity would be inadequate for this objective. It seemed doubtful that this was conducive to identity authenticity—the participant appeared to be conforming to societal expectations to avoid identity threat.

The trans women who participated in this study were of course also living with HIV, another stigmatised element of identity, and thus the perceived need for self-isolation and identity concealment was further compounded by their knowledge that they might also face stigma due to their HIV status. This is outlined next.

HIV Status Concealment and Identity Protection

Interviewees experienced HIV stigma and, thus, exhibited a difficult relationship with their HIV status. None of them expected to test HIV-positive when they did, and most attributed the cause of their infection to the actions of others. Yet, there were also intense feelings of self-blame and self-disgust:

> I kind of blame myself everyday…I just felt the whole world falling. I just, I don't know, I just asked the nurse how long I have to live…I really can't put it in, in words. It's just, it was really negative, that's all I can say, you know.

> I still struggle with it…Yeah, anger at being [HIV-positive]. I still feel stupid for having it…Yeah, so there's a lot of anger, I guess. I mean, I'm not really at peace really with it…I don't feel I can have a sex life with anybody because essentially I just feel contagious.

> I take a lot of drugs and that's just how I cope with it…We all just drown our sorrows in booze and coke.

Individuals clearly experienced threats to identity associated with their HIV diagnosis. Several interviewees harboured significant self-blame and anger due to their HIV infection, which they felt could have been avoided if they had acted differently. Indeed, there was significant regret and guilt among interviewees, many of whom felt that their HIV infection could have been avoided if they were not trans. This was symptomatic of their lack of social support since they were essentially unable to develop a more favourable reconstrual of their experience of becoming HIV-positive and of living with the condition (see Jaspal, Eriksson, & Nynäs, 2020).

The content of the self-stigma was diverse—some metaphorically described their worlds as 'falling' when they learned of their infection, suggesting that the positive diagnosis was life-limiting, if not life-ending. On the other hand, others construed themselves as 'contagious' and, thus, felt unable to have a romantic relationship. In view of the limited HIV knowledge that interviewees had, many were unaware of the benefits of being HIV undetectable for both their own individual health and for public health due to the decreased risk of onward HIV transmission. The lack of awareness of U=U led some to construe themselves as contagious and to conceal this information from other people. They did not wish to be perceived as contagious by other people because they believed that this would expose them to further stigma associated not only with their trans identity but also with their positive serostatus. The coping strategies reported by interviewees were almost entirely maladaptive in that they relied on denying or escaping reality through substance and alcohol misuse, self-isolation and concealment of their HIV status, as several participants outlined:

> I went into this world where nothing else mattered no more because, you know, there was just a lot of sex and drugs and clients but no real talking about me, the real me, or telling anyone I was HIV.

Self-disclosure, that is, talking about the 'real me' was rare in the participant sample, since many simply believed that this was not possible. Due to the challenges in relation to constructing and disclosing their trans identity, some individuals were almost 'primed' to live a life of identity concealment. They reported that they had become accustomed to concealing aspects of their identity during their lives and that this 'felt normal'. Furthermore, there was much trepidation about discussing their lives with others due to a pervasive suspicion about the intentions of others. Some interviewees themselves believed that they had developed an element of paranoia due to previous adverse experiences and that their paranoid thoughts limited their quality of life. On the whole, interviewees did not feel able to share the challenges associated their subsequent HIV diagnosis. The only coping strategies, which they believed to be available to them, were individualised methods of identity concealment.

Accordingly, participants reported little or no access to social support and instead reiterated their preference not to share their HIV status with others:

I have felt like...I'm not quite ready to be out about it, I'm very private about it.

I'm quite a private person when it comes to it so it's like I said you know I- I choose not to talk mm, I mean I've just told you that my- I kind of like cry it away.

I just wish it would go away and while I'm taking the pill, it does sort of go away.

Although the participant (above) described herself as a 'private person', she noted that her alternative strategy for coping—self-isolation—was ineffective as she tended to 'cry it away'. Moreover, the construal of status concealment as reflective of their personality may reflect a long-standing sense of isolation and lack of social connectedness experienced by trans women who are frequently stigmatised and marginalised. Indeed, several interviewees believed that they were alone in the world, emotionally speaking, and that, because others reportedly did not understand their lives, experiences and identities, it was futile to attempt to exchange confidences with them. The strategy of denial (of their HIV status) was facilitated by the fact that they were taking ART and, thus, did not have to think about being HIV-positive due to their generally good health. Although several interviewees felt reliant on themselves (to cope), some also noted that they themselves felt 'unreliable':

I was born alone and that's the way I'm going, you can't count on anyone else to care or help or what have you. But I'm not that reliable myself because sometimes I go and do something stupid and just shock myself... I mean, being HIV and that, it's stupid to just go out on a bender and coked up and let a load of guys have sex with you. That's stupid really.

In exploring why they concealed their HIV status, participants pervasively noted a perceived risk of rejection from others due to their HIV status:

[I'm] scared of being rejected...For me it's scary, because it's hard for me to make friends and that so I'm scared of being rejected but- then other people in the past have tried to- and used my trust and I've learnt from that, and it's- it's always hard to trust people.

My thought was I told people they wouldn't go with me. That they would automatically reject me because I was HIV.

All of the interviewees described adverse experiences of rejection due to other identity elements, such as sexuality and gender, in the past, which had primed them to anticipate rejection. Many were fearful of rejection and sceptical about trusting others. HIV added an additional layer of complexity to their identities, which could lead to further rejection. Indeed, some even described previous experiences of physical violence from romantic partners when they disclosed their HIV status:

> I used to do the right thing but now I do the right thing for me and that's not telling that I'm HIV...a married guy I was with just freaked out and started hitting me, calling me a dirty bitch and hitting me harder and harder because... I was scared for my life, all because I told him I'm HIV.

> The safe option is just not to shout about it...it's his responsibility to stick a condom on. It isn't mine to put myself in that sort of situation.

As observed in previous research, trans women (including those living with HIV) are at increased risk of violence and many report experiences of (sexual) violence. Interviewees had faced violence not only because of their vulnerable position as trans women living in a context in which they perceived themselves to have few rights and limited protection but also because of their HIV status. Several interviewees reported being fearful of disclosing their HIV status because they had been victimised when doing so. Some were accused of trying to pass on HIV intentionally and of putting their partners at risk. Given that they had not disclosed their HIV status to others who might provide support, they also felt uneasy about seeking support in relation to their experiences of victimisation and violence. This essentially created a vicious circle of HIV disclosure to partners, victimisation and the decision not to disclose their HIV status to others for fear of further victimisation and violence.

There was simply a perception that it was safer not to disclose their HIV status to others and, thus, when partners suggested, or insisted on, condomless sex, this presented a dilemma. It is noteworthy that some of the interviewees were not virally suppressed which increased the risk of onward HIV transmission if they did not use a condom. As highlighted in the extracts above, some interviewees resolved this dilemma by referring to their own physical and emotional safety, noting that it was too risky to disclose their status to partners. Furthermore, the responsibility to use condoms was attributed to their partners, rather to themselves, as they constructed themselves as the 'passive partner' both sexually and in terms of power relations between themselves (as trans women) and their more powerful and assertive cisgender male partners.

Yet, some participants did seek support in the form of transient intimacy with sexual partners without disclosing their HIV status to them:

> I just lived my life as normal, I spent quite a bit of time in gay saunas and things so I was sort of sexually active. Didn't really tell very many people that I have HIV I sort of tried to keep that quiet. I thought well I use protection and I use condoms they would never know. It's just- I didn't know how to handle- so how am I going to handle- do I tell the person before we met? And then I- and yeah, it's just- when you just concentrate on yourself first... Scared of being rejected.

In the face of psychological adversity, people of course attempt to cope. Interviewees described their attempts to establish a sense of normality in their lives subsequent to their HIV diagnosis, which, for most, represented a psychologically challenging and aversive experience. The respondent (above) reported having multiple casual sexual partners prior to her diagnosis, many of whom she met in gay saunas. Some of the interviewees reported compartmentalising their HIV status in their minds, that is, to cordon off this information from other aspects of identity. This enabled them to continue to pursue the behaviours that re-established a sense of continuity in their lives and identities. Continuity was necessary for some because their HIV diagnosis represented something deeply negative due partly to unresolved internalised HIV stigma:

> It was just sort of that feeling of being contagious, just that I can't- I can't deal with the rejection of telling somebody, I can't deal with the thought of infecting somebody else and so it was just easier not to.

Participants themselves reported negative characteristics of living with HIV, such as feeling 'contagious' or 'dirty' and, thus, assumed that others would think of them in similar ways. Indeed, most reported first-hand experiences of such stigmatisation from others to whom they disclosed their status. The key point is that internalised HIV stigma appeared to heighten a sense of hypervigilance about how others might react. Some interviewees even found such stigmatisation from others to be reasonable since they made such stigmatising attributions themselves. This led to a preference of identity concealment rather than disclosure.

For some, the strategy of compartmentalising their HIV status (and the consequential strategy of concealing their HIV status from others, including sexual partners) allowed them to continue to meet sexual partners in gay saunas. This in turn enhanced their sense of continuity between past, present and future. Fear of stigma, rejection and discontinuity in identity led individuals to adopt the compartmentalisation and concealment strategies in the face of their HIV diagnosis. They noted that their use of condoms obviated the need to disclose their HIV status to sexual partners but many did also acknowledge their sense of being powerless to insist on condom use with sexual partners who preferred not to use them. The very act of insisting on condom use was perceived as threatening since this could lead to difficult conversations about why condoms were necessary, thereby challenging the efficacy and sustainability of the compartmentalisation and concealment strategies. It is crucial to note that these strategies were, in part, viewed as pivotal for retaining continuity in the face of discontinuity and threatened self-esteem in the face of potential HIV stigma.

There was a recurrent theme in participants' accounts about the need to conceal their HIV status from others due to low levels of trust and the fear of involuntary disclosure of their HIV status. One interviewee reported never disclosing her positive diagnosis to a former romantic partner, which whom she eventually broke up:

> Obviously with the whole cheating drama [with her former partner] and it was bittersweet, because even though we broke up, I have never told him, or he has never come to me, but I know for a fact it's him because there's nobody else that I was with at the time and I'd been with him for four years and he has totally changed, and every time when we would see face-to-face, he has that look on his face like oh- like he's confused so- I have a deep feeling within myself that he knows, but he don't know maybe I do know, I don't know- 'cause obviously I make things look quite normal, but deep down inside I do go through a lot of things, I do think about my future, um right now.

On the one hand, the participant wished to disclose her status to her partner so that he could be tested for HIV and to seek treatment if he was unaware of his HIV status. On the other hand, she was fearful about the consequences of disclosing her HIV status to him because she believed that he might perceive her as the source of his HIV infection and essentially 'blame' her. Indeed, several interviewees described the stigma that they faced when disclosing their HIV status to partners who reportedly blamed their trans partners drawing on stereotypes of trans women being promiscuous and invariably involved in sex work. This can disempower trans women living with HIV from seeking the support that they require (from significant others) in order to cope effectively. Indeed, most interviewees reported struggling to come to terms with their HIV diagnosis and expressed concerns about the future, especially in relation to future relationships. This could be attributed to the pervasive tendency to conceal this information from others, which precluded the derivation of social support.

THE SOCIAL AND ECONOMIC COSTS OF HIV DISCLOSURE

Some individuals believed that disclosure of their HIV status could have adverse social and economic implications for them:

> I just don't feel comfortable having to tell someone that I'm HIV positive at the moment, trust for me is a big thing with people, 'cause I have seen a lot of issues going on with people and trust me, you hear all kinds of people business on the street and I just try and keep my business- I mean for the fact I own a [business], I have to try and keep it up ...I'm trending, I'm on the nineteen- thirty four thousand followers [on social media], I have a good followed [business]- followings- I have to protect what's important to me.

> For a trans woman to come out as positive could be career-ending basically because we get enough stick for being trans so those who make it can kiss it all goodbye if it gets out.

The participants (above) had established and ran their own business. Indeed, several participants believed that disclosure of their HIV status could reflect negatively on their occupational identity, leading some employers to treat them differently or some clients to cease to use their services. One participant construed as her decision to conceal her HIV status from others as a means of 'protecting what's important to me', that is, her business. She clearly believed that disclosure of her traumatic experience of being diagnosed with HIV would imperil her occupational identity. This reflected not only her previous experiences of prejudice when disclosing her status but also her anticipation of societal stigma if she were to do so in the future. Another interviewee noted that, as a trans woman, she was at particularly high risk of stigma and rejection from others due to negative stereotypes of trans people. This was also observable in the sphere of education, given that one interviewee (who was a student) believed that involuntary disclosure of both her trans identity and HIV-positive status might result in her losing her place at university:

> If I tell them I'm positive will they see me as a risk and just throw me out? I don't know these things. In my country, yes, you'd be forced out. I can't risk it so I just stay quiet about it, it's the best thing for me.

On the one hand, the participant drew on negative social representations of trans people and HIV, which were pervasive in her country, leading her to believe that she would face disadvantage in the UK. On the other hand, first-hand personal experiences of stigma from people to whom she had disclosed her identity further compounded these negative social representations, which in turn led her to believe that they also existed in the UK context. She was unaware of legislation designed to protect the rights of minorities, including those of gender minorities and those living with HIV. Her decision to conceal her HIV status and to pursue 'the best thing for me' also deprived her of any possible social support.

Furthermore, due to the size of the trans community, which, for some interviewees, became their principal source of interpersonal support and networking (unrelated to their HIV status), there was a perceived risk of exploitation following HIV status disclosure:

> But yeah, I go there [to a clinic in London] because the centres in Liverpool are- I know girls that y- we know it's a small community when you go out and then people can kind of like use that against you and yeah no so, you know it's just- I don't want to risk it so...It's something that people will always use against you.

> I give you advice, don't create and HIV clinic for- an HIV clinic for transgender people, because we don't want to meet each other at an HIV clinic.

Respondents feared that their HIV status may be used as a 'weapon' against them by others (including by other trans women), that is, that others might 'use that against you'. The 'weaponisation' of HIV has been observed in other populations and is a significant stressor for many people living with HIV (e.g. Gielen et al., 2000). However, it did appear to be especially acute in this participant sample. Indeed, when one participant was informed about the objective of the study, which was to use the research findings to inform clinical practice with trans people at risk of, or living with, HIV, she advised the interviewer not to conclude that trans-specific clinical services were beneficial. This was no criticism of any particular trans-specific services. Indeed, most interviewees reported very favourable experiences in these clinical settings. However, this did reflect an underlying fear of involuntary disclosure of their HIV status—particularly in the trans community. More generally, interviewees recognised the stigma appended to HIV and feared the consequences that this might have for their own identities if their HIV status were involuntarily disclosed to others. They believed that the risk of involuntary disclosure of their HIV status would be high if other trans women were to learn of it. This led some individuals to seek HIV care far away or to delay seeking HIV care altogether:

[The trans specific clinic] is very good. So obviously I go to [the clinic] as a HIV-positive female but really I go to [the clinic] for the transitioning side of life. So it's where I get all my counselling and all my sort of mentoring but yeah so I expect there are other trans women there that are HIV but I don't know because I've never really discussed it with them but I'm sure there must be.

The participant took the active decision to compartmentalise her health-care needs, pursuing those related to her transition in the trans-specific clinic and those relating to her HIV infection in other clinical settings. The compartmentalisation strategy was designed to reduce the risk of involuntary disclosure of her HIV status to other trans service users because the perceived advantages of HIV disclosure reportedly did not outweigh the perceived disadvantages of doing so.

It is noteworthy that most interviewees did in principle acknowledge the potential benefits of sharing their HIV status with trusted others and of deriving social support. However, for most, the risks associated with HIV disclosure were too great. One interviewee described the potential consequences of HIV disclosure for her career as a sex worker:

You have to keep it very private because...many of us are still in sex work...it can ruin someone's professional life basically, because if this- if something like this came out, if someone knew the sex worker- and- and nowadays like especially- it's very much like Trip Advisor because there are forums and people writing reviews about people so if any - any not only

HIV people- any comment on any sexual disease them comes out it will ruin forever this person.

As discussed in Chapter 7, for several interviewees, sex work was the principal source of income and constituted their occupational identity. HIV disclosure was perceived as an existential threat to this identity. They outlined the need for a positive public identity in the world of sex work, often pointing to the significance of other online forums in which trans sex and the services they offer are evaluated. HIV was construed as a 'sexual disease' which could potentially obliterate one's sex worker career and, thus, livelihood. Crucially, interviewees generally observed the limited employment opportunities for trans women. In short, the pursuit of social support was at odds with one's career. Consequently, all of the sex workers in this study refrained from disclosing their HIV status, which precluded access to social support.

At least two interviewees expressed concerns about the risk of physical violence from clients who learned of their positive HIV status, highlighting not only a potential economic threat but also a physical threat:

I have some clients that have really dark backgrounds like you can- like-proper gangsters or whatever and they'll just drop you and yeah well so yeah it's obviously it's dangerous isn't it?

If my clients found out, I'd get beaten up or the phone would be ringing and if someone is HIV-positive because you know, nobody really uses a condom, they'll be knocking on my door harassing me. I don't need that in my life.

As noted above, a participant who was a sex worker reported having disclosed her HIV status to nobody in England and, though resident in Northern England, that she opted to travel to London to receive HIV care in order to reduce the risk of involuntary disclosure of her status. She believed that she would be at risk of physical violence, or even death, if her clients, whom she described as 'proper gangsters', were to learn of her positive serostatus. Such fears often precluded HIV disclosure—to co-workers, friends or family members—and thus social support. In most cases, concealment of one's HIV status constituted a strategy for coping with threat but, in this participant's case, it was also deemed essential for survival as a trans sex worker. Similarly, other interviewees believed that, by disclosing their HIV status to others, their clients might come to know of this and engage in blame attribution, that is, to blame them for 'spreading HIV'. The trans women who participated in this study generally reported a sense of hypervigilance and regarded themselves as 'an easy target' for blame attribution because they were trans and sex workers. Consequently, they refrained from disclosing their HIV status to others and opted for identity concealment and self-isolation.

OVERVIEW

This chapter focuses on the coping responses of trans women living with HIV who face multiple layers of stigma. In view of the pervasive sense of hypervigilance in relation to the intentions of others, interviewees reported resorting to individualised strategies for coping with identity threat, such as identity concealment and self-isolation. Individuals felt uncomfortable about disclosing aspects of their identity to others because they feared exposure to further stigma, prejudice and hostility. They were distrustful of others because previous experiences had demonstrated that this was the safest type of thinking for them. This type of coping essentially deprived them of social support networks which ordinarily enable people to cope more effectively with identity threat. Yet, the anticipated costs of self-disclosure were deemed to outweigh the potential advantages of doing so. Although designed to protect the self-esteem and continuity principles of identity, identity concealment and self-isolation could undermine people's sense of identity authenticity, since they may feel obliged to present themselves in inauthentic ways and, thus, unable to 'be themselves'. Crucially, in their quest to conceal their identity from others, individuals were also deprived of informational networks that might enable them to inform themselves and, thus, cope more effectively. In particular, trans women living with HIV may be especially fearful of self-disclosure to other trans women given that there appears to be decreased interpersonal trust and a sense that others will 'weaponise' their HIV status. Involuntary disclosure of one's HIV status was deemed to be especially harmful to one aspect of identity, namely one's occupational identity as a trans sex worker. This is discussed in the next chapter.

References

Breakwell, G. M. (1986). *Coping with threatened identities*. London: Methuen.

Gielen, A. C., Fogarty, L., O'Campo, P., Anderson, J., Keller, J., & Faden, R. (2000). Women living with HIV: Disclosure, violence, and social support. *Journal of Urban Health, 77*(3), 480–491. https://doi.org/10.1007/BF0 2386755.

Jaspal, R. (2014). Sexuality, migration and identity among gay Iranian migrants to the UK. In Y. Taylor & R. Snowdon (Eds.), *Queering religion, religious queers* (pp. 44–60). London: Routledge.

Jaspal, R., Eriksson, P., & Nynäs, P. (2020). Coping with HIV: Accounts from gay men living with HIV in Finland. Under review.

CHAPTER 7

Sex Work and HIV

Abstract Most of the participants in the EXTRA Study reported previous
or current engagement in sex work. In this chapter, first, the psychologically aversive aspects of engaging in sex work as a trans woman living with
HIV are described. This includes exposure to negative stereotypes, stigma
and hostility from others. Second, the risks to psychological health, sexual
health and physical wellbeing associated with sex work are described.
Third, the coping strategies in relation to identity threat related to sex
work are examined. On the one hand, sex work can threaten self-esteem
due to the pervasive social stigma appended to it but, on the other hand,
it can enhance self-efficacy given that trans women may achieve financial
autonomy.

Keywords Sex work · Self-efficacy · HIV risk · Identity management

The Psychological Burden of Sex Work

Most of the participants had some experience of sex work and three
reported continued engagement in sex work as their principal source of
income. There were many psychologically challenging aspects of sex work
as a trans person living with HIV. Most interviewees acknowledged the
negative stereotypes of trans women and the assumption that they invariably were, or had been, sex workers. Although most of them reported

© The Author(s) 2020
R. Jaspal, *Trans Women and HIV*,
https://doi.org/10.1007/978-3-030-57545-8_7

some experience of sex work, they lamented the automatic assumption that they were sex workers because of their transness. This was challenging for self-esteem and reportedly made some people feel ashamed:

> There's a lingering belief that we sell our bodies, that trans bodies are just for the enjoyment of cis people, to be looked at, perved on. I feel shame because I have been there.

> I pass, as you can see, and it's good treatment [from other people] but the minute you say you're trans, it's like 'have you been with guys for money?' They don't always say it but you can see that's what they're thinking.

> I resent this idea that trans equals prostitute. It gives people an excuse to treat us like scum.

Interviewees construed the stereotype that equated trans identity with sex work as threatening for identity. They noted that this stereotype, which was uncritically accepted by other (cisgender) people, made them feel ashamed because they acknowledged their own engagement in sex work. This amounted to a threat to self-esteem. There was an element of hypervigilance in that interviewees anticipated, or suspected, that others endorsed this stereotype of trans women, regardless of what they actually said. One of the interviewees reported knowing that this was what others were thinking about trans women. There was some evidence in the interviews of individuals 'analysing' what others were saying in order to detect whether or not they believed that all trans women were sex workers. This suggested that there was some concern about self-presentation and indeed, as demonstrated below, some interviewees went to great lengths to prove to others that they were not sex workers. They wished to protect their continuity of self-presentation as *non*-sex workers.

There was a belief that this stereotype facilitated the mistreatment of trans women, that is, their objectification as 'bodies' which 'are just there for the enjoyment of cis people'. Indeed, one participant noted that others deemed it appropriate to treat trans women 'like scum' because of the assumption that they were sex workers. Furthermore, another interviewee noted that most cisgender people believe that trans women are 'fucked up' and, thus, 'getting up to all sorts'—a reference to engagement in sex work as a strategy for coping with psychological adversity. As noted in previous chapters, the stereotype regarding sex work reflected an overarching stigma of trans women, which was challenging for self-esteem.

It must also be observed that some interviewees were especially perturbed by the social stigma appended to sex work because of their HIV status. More specifically, some had internalised the stigma that they encountered which in turn reinforced the stigma of their HIV status. They believed that they had contracted HIV during the course of, and as a result of, sex work, which was aversive for the self-esteem principle of identity. For some, this gave rise to feelings of guilt and regret, with some wishing that they had never 'given into the stereotype':

> I look back and think 'why was I so stupid?' I wish I'd never given into the stereotype... of being trans and being a prostitute and that. I just played right into this and ended up ruining my life. I feel like such a idiot, like I deserve it or something.

Some interviewees deeply regretted engaging in sex work which they perceived as the source, or cause, of their HIV infection. This led some individuals to experience low self-esteem—the interviewee above felt 'like such an idiot' and that she 'deserved' her HIV infection. In order to cope, some participants attempted to distance sex work from their identity and, in doing so, themselves stigmatised trans female sex workers:

> The fact of sleeping with different- different people, and not only that like, I don't know, like I kind of grown up in a Christian home as well where they say your body's a temple, so I still have that in me as to- you could be who you are but respect- self-respect and dignity is something you carry a long way and that... It is very easy because what the trans industry- I would say industry, let's use that phrase, what the trans community is promoting on social media and promoting to others is trans women have this.

> It's easy to just sell your body and make some money that way but try doing what I've done, now that's hard. I've always stuck up for the trans community and, you know, just make some money so you can get your Louis Vuitton handbag or what not, it's sad.

> It's the low intelligence to get up and do other stuff. I get that some have the pressure but it's the easy way out.

Many recognised the stereotype of trans women as sex workers and most interviewees acknowledged some first-hand experience of sex work in the past. Yet, as demonstrated in these extracts, there was a pervasive desire for positive distinctiveness in the participant sample. Individuals contrasted their own decision to disengage from sex work with the apparently superficial reasons that other trans women reportedly continue to engage in sex work. As indicated in the extracts, one participant constructed herself as having 'self-respect and dignity' while another attributed sex work to the desire to purchase expensive goods, such as designer brand handbags. Furthermore, some interviewees depicted trans women who engage in sex work as being less intelligent than those who do not, although they did generally acknowledge the potential pressures that one might face as a trans person (living with HIV). Crucially, by constructing trans women who engage in sex work as vain, lazy and devoid of self-respect, interviewees presented themselves as positively distinctive from them. This reflected an 'us versus them' dynamic, which has also been referred to as downward comparison (Wills, 1981).

More generally, it appeared that some participants acknowledged, had internalised and uncritically accepted the negative stereotype of trans women as sex workers, from which they wished to distance themselves. Indeed, some referred to 'the trans industry', suggesting that there was a commercialisation of transness and trans bodies, which was attributed to trans women themselves rather than to external pressures. The key point is that some interviewees positioned themselves outside of this category (i.e. the trans industry), which suggested that they were different from 'most' trans women. This positive distinctiveness also facilitated a sense of self-esteem, since participants were able to highlight positive characteristics of their own identity (e.g. self-respect and dignity) which they 'evidenced' by not engaging in sex work. Thus, in order to resist stigma at an individual level, some interviewees internalised and reproduced negative stereotypes of 'most' trans women, positioning themselves as being positively distinctive from them:

The promotion and the way that now that you have social media there's Instagram pages that escorting- inviting you to become an escort, just girls that I know that I grew up with that would leave the Netherlands and go to Switzerland and go to New York and go to Miami and just go on escorting and even London they come and they do escorting and they make mad money but at the end of the day, what- as I say to them what have you done to better yourself? And that is like, you're waiting for your next fix, your next client and I always say you're the new girl today, but there's a new girl tomorrow and the day after and the day after and then what's gonna happen you're just gonna end up in a situation, in a predicament that you don't wanna be in, you know, I have respect for everyone, if that's what you wanna do, toodles to you but I have more respect for those that do it, get out of it and do something with their lives, I think that's more, okay cool.

As noted in this extract, trans sex workers were attributed stigmatising characteristics, such as drug use, and it was assumed that they had done nothing to 'better themselves'. The participant was suggesting that trans sex workers did not make the most of their lives and apparently took an easier route than those who 'get out of it and do something with their lives'. She acknowledged having engaged in sex work in the past but had now established her own business. Thus, in essence, she was contrasting her own experience of emerging from the world of sex work with trans women who decide to persevere as sex workers. Her own experience was constructed as being more challenging but also more rewarding and fruitful than that of current sex workers, which enabled her to derive a sense of positive distinctiveness from other trans women who engage in sex work.

Those interviewees who reproduced the stigma of sex work and distanced themselves from it were also invited to describe their own first-hand experiences of engaging in sex work. They mainly acknowledged initial temptation due to the perceived financial lucrativeness but subsequent regret and guilt:

If I want something, see something, do something I will do it, so that what kinda pushed me to become independent financially, yeah, in my way of growing up, I'm gonna be honest, has prostituting cross my mind? Of course, 'cause other friends, other girls does it and that's easy money, but then what hit me is like, can I do it?

I've tried it, I have signed-up online and tried escorting and my first client was this huge guy and he was just ugh, and I was like I can't do this... I was trembling and I just couldn't do it, so pretty much I guess my experience- my first experience kind of was a plus to the reason why I never got in to that field so.

I felt dirty after my first one. He treated me like I am just to be used by him and that's my only purpose. I did it but then hated it and cried for a while. I did it a few more times after but it was making me rich but not making me happy. I was getting depressed with myself.

Interviewees noted the difficulties they experienced in securing employment due to the stigma that they faced and the 'norm' of sex work among trans women, which led them to consider this as a potential career option. They noted that sex work was quite salient as a career option for trans women with several social media pages existing to entice them into this line of work. Moreover, all of the participants had trans friends who were sex workers and who appeared to be earning a satisfactory living. However, they generally reported being less aware of the challenging aspects of sex work (see next section) before embarking upon this career themselves and noted that the 'image' of sex work had been a favourable one for them. They often contrasted this positive image of sex work with the limited employment opportunities that they perceived.

For some participants, their negative initial experiences of sex work led them to disengage from this line of work. There was wide agreement that sex work was difficult because some of the clients were not sexually attractive or desirable to them, which could make it impossible to have sex with them. As indicated in one account, engagement in sex work could also be challenging at a psychological level because of clients' behaviour which some interviewees found demeaning and stigmatising. The pervasive stigma surrounding sex work and the limited sense of choice in this line of work was threatening for identity. Yet, this did present a dilemma for individuals who nevertheless recognised the financial incentive to engage in sex work.

One participant who grew up in difficult socio-economic conditions in Brazil attributed her engagement in sex work to the financial 'escape' that this offered her, as a trans woman:

> I knew I was going to go- sex work, because it is- it is not beautiful to say but, for, for poor people, it is quite a good amount of financial escape- it is, yes it works, if you're poor and you're looking for a way to- yeah. It's very difficult, you know, it's very difficult to get out of poverty on- on conventional routes.

> Being a prostitute was what gave me my independence so I'm glad I did it. It put me through a lot, yeah, but it was what made me an independent woman because I could do what I wanted and I wasn't relying on no one.

For some, sex work was an escape not only from poverty but also from economic and social dependence on others. It provided a means of restoring self-efficacy amid dependence on significant others who were unsympathetic to their desire to transition. Moreover, participants acknowledged the difficulty of an escape through 'conventional routes' for trans women, marginalised from society. This did present a dilemma, however—they were aware of the challenges that lay ahead and the risks associated with sex work (especially violence from clients) but were willing to accept these challenges due to their desire for escapism. Sex work could provide financial, social and psychological freedom from other people who were stigmatising towards their trans identity. Indeed, interviewees often reported that their previous experiences of identity disclosure (or coming out as trans) had been difficult and that, in some cases, they had been given an ultimatum by their parents and significant others: either to 'be normal' (i.e. to conform to the norms associated with the gender they were assigned at birth) or to leave. Sex work facilitated a departure from this situation but presented its own risks and challenges.

Furthermore, for some interviewees, the lure of sex work was compounded by a strong sex drive and a desire for intimacy during early adulthood. In reflecting on their decision to engage in sex work, some noted that the advantages of sex work simply seemed to outweigh the possible risks and challenges:

It was easy back then because I was very young and- and the hormones weren't super high so I was already- I would consider myself to be a sex addict until a few years ago and then when I really got tired of it then I-didn't- want to know any more about it but before then it wasn't- yes-it was sex all day every day basically, sometimes not only for payments, sometimes for fun, yes but yes- sex was really, really present in my life throughout I think ten years.

I think I was doing sex work not just for the money but also because you know it was the time I had with another person and the sex was good and I think it made me feel good for a bit. it was tiring but it filled me in an emotional sense too sort of.... I was going through a lot.

For most of the interviewees, sex work did constitute, or had constituted, a source of income and an occupational identity. Yet, for some, it also represented a type of coping strategy in relation to other adverse events and experiences in their lives. Some reported having a sex addition and noted that sex work addressed this psychological need in addition to providing a living. There were also accounts of previous psychological distress, especially relating to loneliness and isolation, which was alleviated by engaging in intimate sexual encounters with clients during the course of their work. Notwithstanding the challenging aspects of sex work, interviewees reported the inability to derive transient feelings of intimacy with some of their clients, which was psychologically fulfilling. This did present a dilemma, however, since interviewees reported knowing that these bouts of intimacy were transient and short-lived and that sex work entailed risks to their health and wellbeing.

Enforced Risk in Sex Work

Participants described the lucrativeness of a career in sex work, compared to gay male sex workers who reportedly earned much less than trans female sex workers. There was much discussion among interviewees about the various factors that they had considered before embarking upon a career in sex work. They were all aware of the significant social stigma appended to sex work but, in most cases, sex work was construed as providing a sense of self-efficacy.

Yet, the lucrativeness of this career path did lead some trans women to engage in behaviours that they knew could undermine their wellbeing in one way or another. Thus, there was a paradoxical acknowledgement of decreased self-efficacy in sex work—on the one hand, it provided financial independence but, on the other hand, they acknowledged having to engage in non-volitional risks. For instance, high-risk sex, to which participants attributed the cause of their HIV infection, was often perceived to be a standard expectation for trans sex workers:

> I allowed – I did really high-risk things for the money... I'll be with a client and they'll say 'yeah, I'll give you fifty quid [British pounds] if you know, I could take you bareback' and I would say 'yeah, go on then'. To me, it's just, I don't know, it's 50 quid.

> I had quite a reputation for it and, yeah, had a really, I mean I still do, that reputation still follows me and it's on that's hard to shake, because yeah, and loads of drugs, lots of high-risk stuff really and that's it, yeah... All my loyal customers, they look for a very special kind of thing that very few people offer.

Participants who engaged in sex work described pressure from clients to engage in high-risk sex, such as condomless sex and drug use, in exchange for money. Some reported prioritising the financial benefits of sex work over their sexual health, despite being aware of the risks involved. They noted that they had thought about sexual health issues and were aware of the risk of HIV infection associated with condomless sex, but felt pressured to engage in this behaviour because of the financial incentives. Indeed, most interviewees discussed the high expenses that they had as trans women, such as having to spend money on their physical appearance and paying for expensive accommodation. It appeared that the issue of sexual heath was simply relegated to a less prominent position in their thinking.

Although for some participants transient engagement in condomless sex was deemed to be 'part of the job' and could sometimes yield greater payment from clients than sex with condoms, others noted that their 'reputation' was constructed primarily on the basis of their willingness to forego condoms in sex. Indeed, one participant described her reputation for engaging in high-risk sex, from which she benefitted financially given that her 'loyal customers' were often willing to pay more to obtain her services. On the other hand, she acknowledged the risks associated with her sexual behaviour, which continued to imperil her sexual health, but felt unable to disassociate herself from this long-standing reputation and, thus, from engagement in high-risk behaviour. Condomless sex was construed as a marker of distinctiveness as she was reportedly one of the few trans sex workers willing to provide these services. High-risk sex became an aspect of identity as a sex worker and an expectation from clients who solicited her services. Therefore, the participant became financially reliant on it. Several interviewees noted that condomless sex was frequently being requested and expected by customers, which led them to acquiesce:

> I've had clients who say 'turn over' and I take out a condom and they laugh and say 'I'm the one paying you here' so I feel a bit powerless because you're pleasing the customer.

> I just feel that I can't say 'no'. How am I going to pay my rent if he walks off? I thought I'm not going to be that unlucky to end up positive.

These extracts clearly demonstrated the occupational pressures that some trans sex workers face, given that there may be a coercive expectation that they submit to the sexual desires of their clients, notwithstanding the potential risks to their sexual health. The risk of losing clients and, thus, one's livelihood was deemed to be more significant than the comparably small risk of acquiring HIV. Indeed, individuals reported minimising this risk and attempting to convince themselves that they would not be 'unlucky'. More generally, some perceived it as their occupational duty to 'please the customer' and, thus, submitted to sex that they did not desire or that they knew was unsafe.

In addition to the sexual health risks related to sex work, there were risks to psychological wellbeing among sex workers due to perceived pressure to engage in undesirable sexual behaviour:

> I'm passive[1] but for work you have- I have to be active, it's just the way it works you have to adapt to the situation and you have to do things you don't even like in the sex industry... It's only going to work if you, you know, make an effort, so making an effort was also top, to top...so I was taking testosterone drops and Viagra at the same time which is a great contradiction. My doctors really wouldn't understand it. They say 'I can't take you seriously on your gender reassignment request if you are taking Viagra and if you are having sex on- on- on a top position.

Although some interviewees accepted the perceived requirements of sex work and resigned themselves to the reality of this line of work, they also discussed the psychologically aversive aspects of sex work. One participant who preferred to be sexually receptive felt obliged to perform the sexually active role with clients who requested this, which she described as 'making an effort'. In order to perform this role satisfactorily, she was compelled to use testosterone and Viagra, which in turn caused challenges with her gender transition. Healthcare professionals were unable to understand her rationale for using testosterone and Viagra simultaneously and for performing the insertive role in sex, which meant that she often had to justify her actions—sometimes unsuccessfully. It has been noted that trans women may feel obliged to 'prove' their transness by conforming to binary gender norms and living in accordance with the gender with which their identity (Pearce, 2018). Yet, sex workers may be compelled by clients to engage in sexual behaviours which they themselves do not desire or which may be construed by others (such as healthcare professionals) as being inconsistent with the gender into which they are transitioning. This can present dilemmas. In short, there was a perceived clash between the responsibilities associated with her occupational

---

[1] The term 'active' is used to refer to the insertive sexual partner, while 'passive' refers to the receptive sexual partner.

identity as a sex worker and the social psychological aspects of her identity as a sexually receptive trans woman. This appeared to be constructed as a threat to psychological coherence.

Furthermore, interviewees noted a series of other potential sexual risk behaviours in which they felt compelled to engage as a result of their occupational identity. They perceived limited agency and control over the behaviours that were reportedly demanded by clients:

If I do prostitution I have to take drugs because of the clients.

Oral sex isn't an option, it's just like- there is- it's a sort of rule, when you receive phone calls they will ask and if you say 'no I only do protected oral sex' you're just not going to get a good result, and you have to make a lot of investment, so you have to cover your expenses and make a profit and it's only going to work if you, you know.

There's no 'shall we go gentle'. It is 'this is how I want it because this is costing me'. Sometimes I don't like it but it's what you do in this game, to survive.

As demonstrated in the interview extracts above, sex workers may be compelled to engage in drug use and oral sex 'because of the clients'. Some of the interviewees differentiated between different types of sexual behaviour—some were deemed to be 'part of the job' while others were construed as more intimate and appropriate only to romantic relationships. Several described oral sex as a type of sexual behaviour in which they were willing to engage only with a romantic partner, such as a boyfriend, rather than with clients. Yet, they did not feel able to negotiate the type of sex that they were having with clients. Furthermore, as another participant noted, the pressure to engage in undesirable, risky sexual behaviours was further reinforced by clients who reminded trans sex workers that they were paying for sex. The participant's observation that her compliance with clients' demands enabled her 'to survive' was a reference to interviewees' financial reliance on sex work and the economic difficulties that could ensue from non-compliance with clients' demands.

In addition to the sexual risks associated with sex work, there was elaborate discussion about the risk of physical violence from clients and other men during the course of their work. This was clearly unsettling for interviewees who nevertheless felt obliged to endure this risk in order to survive:

That was tough, every week there was blood, not mine I was very lucky, because I was the only one on my street that was working safe method, because the other girls they weren't working really, they were just pretending they were working but they wanted to steal, so they had clients that well, got stolen they were very upset, they wanted to be the first one that they would find because they won't find the same girl because they knew how to do it, they would change the wig, they would change the dress and then they wouldn't be able to find them so yeah sometimes they would just like run us through or throw rocks at us and things, so that was difficult I was very lucky to come out of it in one piece.

Sex workers operate in a complex environment. As participants noted, some sex workers themselves engage in behaviours that can put the well-being of other sex workers at risk. Interviewees who engaged in sex work described being victimised randomly by angry clients, which rendered the work environment a risky and hostile one. This was described as a significant hazard in the workplace which was simply accepted as part of the job. Yet, the psychological impact for several interviewees who described such hostile work conditions was considerable—they described fear, anxiety and hypervigilance. Some also highlighted the relief that they felt when they returned home after work because of the heightened state of anxiety that they experienced during the course of their work. Participants reported developing several strategies for attempting to manage their anxiety but this remained a distressing activity. There were several first-hand accounts of violence, which continued to cause psychological distress even as participants recalled their experiences, even though some were no longer sex workers:

There was one guy that pulled a knife at me and he was just a psychopath because he didn't steal me and I thought well, I'm sorry because if he was stealing me I'd just give him money and that's okay I go home, it has worked before but no he wasn't- he was a sadist basically and I was yeah, I was really scared and I... and he got very upset and ... then I jumped through the window.

Sometimes you get beaten and if you tell the police they will just laugh in your face or maybe just ask you stupid questions about being trans. I didn't want to tell anyone. I just took it all because it was what you have to do.... one guy knew I'm positive. He didn't have sex. He just did things to me, abusing me, paying me. It was because I had HIV and the girls told him this. I still have nightmares about him and it's marked my life.

Respondents recounted psychologically traumatic experiences of violence during the course of their work. One participant noted that she had encountered people who had no intention of soliciting sexual services or of robbing sex workers but who just wished to perpetrate violence against them. Some attributed these experiences to their vulnerable position as trans sex workers in that they believed that they were easy targets for sadists and that they had no recourse to the authorities who were reportedly unsympathetic when they did file a complaint.

Furthermore, one participant attributed her experience of sexual violence to her status as a trans sex worker *living with HIV*. She believed that her HIV status rendered her more vulnerable to such acts of violence because she was deemed to be of decreased worth compared to others. Like many other interviewees, she decided not to report this incident to the police because she did not believe that she would be taken seriously, as a trans sex worker. The experience continued to haunt her psychologically. Many interviewees were concerned that they themselves might be arrested for sex work if they were to be complain and that their HIV status might be involuntarily disclosed to others if they were to engage with the police.

Overall, it was evident that sex work exposed interviewees to a variety of risks—to their sexual health, physical safety and psychological health—but that they felt compelled to endure these risks as a normal part of their work life. Furthermore, when difficulties did arise in the workplace, such as exposure to physical violence, the vast majority were unable or unwilling to report these incidents to the police because they clearly had a low level of institutional trust. They believed that institutions, such as the police, were not supportive of trans women (living with HIV) and that they might experience greater adversity if they were to attempt to derive support from these reportedly cisgenderist institutions.

Managing Identity as a Sex Worker

The experience of being trans, HIV-positive and a sex worker can be psychologically challenging. As indicated above, these multiple layers of stigma can cause multiple threats to identity. The data clearly indicated that individuals were attempting to cope. Coping occurred on at least two levels: first, there was a need to cope at a psychological level and, second, individuals were mindful of their public image and, thus, managed their public identity carefully to ensure that this did not undermine their career as sex workers.

Interviewees described a variety of strategies to cope with the stigma associated with sex work and to protect self-esteem:

> When I was in Brazil at home. I went out and worked the streets and came home and when I was home, I was not trans, not HIV, not a prostitute. I put it out of my head and that was OK. It worked for me for a while but I was not true to myself.... At night, I went out and I wasn't doing anything to show who I am at home.

> I didn't think about being positive when I was working. If someone asked I said 'no' because it was true for me. I just didn't think of it, like a trance.

> I knew it was dirty but I had to separate this out and just not think about it because I had the big thing about being trans all my life, being gay, now getting HIV, and it was all a bit too much for me, so I just didn't think about being a prostitute on top of that.

Participants reported having to conceal their career as sex workers from significant others due to the anticipation of stigma and rejection from them. Some of them described leading a double life and meticulously guarding their secret from significant others. This was psychologically taxing since there was a need to conceal, lie and retain credibility in the eyes of others. There was concern not only about involuntary disclosure of their gender identity and HIV status but also of their career as sex workers. The needed to lie and ensuring that the lie was not revealed was reportedly overwhelming for some interviewees.

In order to protect their identity at this interpersonal level, some participants also reported enacting intrapsychic coping strategies. As noted in the extracts, some interviewees compartmentalised their career as a sex worker from other aspects of their identity, confining sex work to 'the streets' and not to the home environment. They simply did not think about sex work or their career as a sex worker while at home, thereby creating a protective 'barrier' around this information so that it did not gain access to consciousness in the 'wrong' context, that is, at home. In other words, this reflected an attempt to ensure that knowledge of one's sex work was confined to the external environment and that one's family members were not able to access this information.

Similarly, interviewees reported the challenges to self-esteem posed by knowledge of their HIV status, which led them to conceal this information from others but also to suppress knowledge of their HIV status at a psychological level. While engaging in sex work, participants no longer thought about their HIV status, which was described by one individual 'like a trance' in that this information did not gain access to consciousness. As demonstrated earlier in this volume, many of the interviewees had not fully come to terms with their HIV diagnosis and experienced threats to their sense of self-esteem. Some felt 'dirty'—a feeling that was compounded by the experience of occupying multiple stigmatised positions, such as being trans and a sex worker. By compartmentalising their HIV status from their career as sex workers, they were no longer required to think about the potential implications of being a trans sex worker living with a communicable virus. They no longer experienced decreased self-esteem due to their HIV status and did not need to think about self-care behaviours or behaviours that might reduce the risk of onward HIV transmission to clients.

Another strategy used by participants to cope with the social stigma appended to sex work was to reject this stigma. Most interviewees described the very difficult circumstances under which trans people became sex workers, noting the prejudice against them in the workplace, which reportedly reduced their employment opportunities:

A lot of people say being a prostitute is dirty or you've got no morals or whatever but I see it as a survival strategy because where was I going to get work being trans? Who was going to employ me? Society rejects me and you have to do something.

The respondent rejected the stigma of sex work (i.e. its status as a 'dirty' occupation practised by those with 'no morals') by re-construing sex work as 'a survival strategy'. This was attributed to the societal rejection of trans people and to the exclusion of trans people from the workplace, which reportedly compelled them to resort to sex work. By re-construing sex work as a survival strategy, the interviewee attributed responsibility to a transphobic society. This in turn enabled some individuals to deflect the stigma which, if accepted, could have deleterious implications for self-esteem. Compartmentalisation and denial represented common strategies for coping with the stigma of sex work, which might otherwise challenge self-esteem.

Moreover, there were attempts to manage one's identity as a sex worker in self-presentation to clients to ensure that individuals were able to construct a self-image characterised by esteem and thereby attract suitable clients:

> We have basically a reviews section and people can say 'she's good' or 'she's shit' and it makes a big difference because you get good clients and good money when your reviews are good.

> You know, it's like you're being judged and rated literally. Seeing a bad rating would plunge me into thinking 'am I worth it? am I shit?'

> Yes, only if you're trying to build a reputation, which I did and it worked out really well for me because I was- I mean yeah super feminine and beautiful and well taken care of, and I wouldn't rush and I would refuse clients if I had- if was tired, if I just had a couple or a few and then I'll just say no because I didn't want to… I was that careful about not getting bad reviews, some girls weren't and they'd pay the price, because once you start getting bad reviews you- you'll notice it, I think, you notice the quality and the amount of clients you're getting.

Interviewees expressed concern about the reviews that they might receive from clients given the perceived importance of these reviews in determining their job security as sex workers. The nature of the reviews was perceived to influence the quality and quantity of clients. As noted above, this in turn meant that sex workers were able to be more selective about their clients and to refuse services to undesirable clients or to clients who demanded undesirable sexual activities.

Some interviewees also noted the psychological impact of negative reviews in terms of self-esteem and self-efficacy. On the one hand, negative reviews might limit the scope and effectiveness of one's career as a sex worker. Furthermore, in view of the perception of sex work as a passage to greater autonomy, independence and competence in life, threats to one's career as a sex worker amounted to a threat to the self-efficacy principle of identity. It is also important to note that several interviewees describe their intense efforts to 'build a reputation' in their career as sex workers, which had taken time. This was empowering for individuals since it constituted an example of success in their lives, which provided feelings of both self-efficacy and self-esteem. On the other hand, most interviewees reported vulnerability in relation to self-esteem, principally because their lives had been characterised by self-doubt, shame and identity concealment, especially in relation to their transness. Negative reviews in relation to one's performance as a sex worker could undermine the already vulnerable self-esteem principle of identity because some came to internalise the negative characteristics attributed to them by clients in their online reviews.

Participants' concerns about negative reviews were further aggravated by their fear of involuntary disclosure of their HIV status:

> I'm known for a service I offer and so I can't be having people finding out that I'm positive because then my service is going to be like less, customers won't want it. Now they do.

Earlier in this chapter, it was noted that one of the participants believed that her mistreatment at the hands of her client could be attributed to her HIV status in that she believed that HIV stigma enabled her client to mistreat and abuse her. Similarly, other interviewees believed that involuntary disclosure of their HIV status could result in adverse outcomes for their occupational identity (and self-efficacy) as sex workers. They predicted that fewer clients would be interested in frequenting an HIV-positive sex worker and, as indicated in Chapter 6, that they may face violence from clients who learned of their HIV status.

Positive self-presentation was especially important because a poor public image could undermine one's career as a sex worker, particularly in the digital age of online reviews. Given the important benefits of sex work for self-efficacy—in some cases, enabling trans women to become financially stable and independent—the prospect of career failure posed significant threats to this principle of identity, in particular.

OVERVIEW

In this chapter, the psychological challenges of engaging in sex work were described, focusing on the stigma associated with this occupational identity and the internalisation of this stigma among some individuals. This can be aversive for the self-esteem principle of identity. Some felt unable to disclose their sex worker identity to others. Threats to identity were compounded by the perceived obligation to engage in behaviours that they found risky or undesirable because their clients required them to do so. This was also challenging for the self-efficacy principle of identity since individuals felt unable to refuse. Yet, for many respondents, sex work was also construed as enhancing self-efficacy because it enabled them to achieve financial independence and autonomy in the absence of other vocational opportunities. This presented a dilemma for some interviewees. Identity management as a sex worker was deemed to be important to excel in this line of work—many were uneasy about disclosing their HIV status to potential clients and were concerned about negative reviews, undermining their public identity in the context of sex work. As trans women living with HIV, sex work added an additional layer of complexity to their threatened identities.

References

Pearce, R. (2018). *Understanding trans health: Discourse, power and possibility.* Bristol: Policy Press.

Wills, T. A. (1981). Downward comparison principles in social psychology. *Psychological Bulletin, 90*(2), 245–271. https://doi.org/10.1037/0033-2909.90.2.245.

PART III

Conclusion

CHAPTER 8

Supporting Trans Women Living with HIV

Abstract In this chapter, the social psychological aspects of trans women's experiences of living with HIV are examined. Through the lens of the Health Adversity Risk Model, the multifaceted experiences of stigma, the tendency to self-isolate and to conceal identity aspects, and the challenges of sex work as a trans woman living with HIV are explored. The theoretical, empirical and practical implications of the EXTRA Study are discussed and future research directions are outlined.

Keywords Social psychology · Health Adversity Risk Model · Coping with HIV · Stigma · Identity processes

Social Psychological Perspectives

This volume provides social psychological perspectives on the experiences of trans women living with HIV in the UK. This is important because it is clear that the minority stressors that they face operate at multiple levels—some are socio-structural, while others are psychological. Some trans women report lifelong exposure to structural violence, such as societal stigma, and resort to accepting this stigma uncritically at a psychological level. What is experienced in one's social context may be accepted or resisted at a psychological level. Stigma is a good example. Some trans women living with HIV appear to accept and internalise the stigma that

© The Author(s) 2020
R. Jaspal, *Trans Women and HIV*,
https://doi.org/10.1007/978-3-030-57545-8_8

they encounter, while others may actively resist it. Understanding how and why this may occur is vitally important, since the ability to resist stigma and to cope with it effectively is central to psychological well-being. In accordance with the social psychological approach taken in this volume, it is explicitly acknowledged that people cope at multiple levels of human interdependence. Some coping strategies (such as denial) operate only in the mind of the individual. Others require modifications to one's relationships with other individuals or with other groups. In this volume, there is an attempt to describe the complex myriad of coping strategies available to, and deployed by, trans women living with HIV.

It must be noted that trans women living with HIV are constructing their identity—consisting of multiple elements—within a particular social context which has its own set of norms, values and ideologies. They must confront these norms, values and ideologies and consider how their self-presentation fits within this social context. It would be short-sighted to construct a narrative of identity, wellbeing and behaviour among trans women focusing exclusively on the individual psychological level of analysis—the social context must not only be acknowledged but also woven into our descriptions, explanations and predictors of identity, wellbeing and behaviour.

In this volume, various theoretical frameworks have been described, including the coming out models, minority stress theory, the concept of structural violence and identity process theory. Tenets of all of these models are useful in enhancing our understanding of trans women's experiences of living with HIV. However, when used in isolation, some of these perspectives may provide only a partial account of the experience of living with HIV among trans women. For instance, the coming out process may be complicated by an HIV diagnosis, which may reinforce existing internalised homophobia. Furthermore, in view of the insidious effects of HIV stigma, a positive diagnosis may further challenge individuals' ability to derive pride on the basis of their trans identity, instead opting for identity concealment and isolation. On the other hand, minority stress theory does not fully articulate how and why particular stressors (such as being trans, HIV-positive) challenge psychological wellbeing.

Data from the EXTRA Study suggest that these stressors operate in complex ways, potentially threatening identity in some contexts but enhancing it in others. Tenets of these theoretical frameworks therefore form the basis of the adapted version of the Health Adversity Risk Model, which is applied to data derived from the EXTRA Study.

Describing and Predicting Risk

Consistent with the Health Adversity Risk Model, it is indicated that trans women living with HIV respond to identity threat (associated with exposure to structural violence and other stressors) using various coping strategies—some of which are adaptive and others which are maladaptive. In this volume, it has been demonstrated that they face multi-layered stigma in relation to various identity elements (e.g. being trans, HIV-positive, a former or current sex worker), that further psychological challenges may be experienced in attempting to reconcile sex work and a positive HIV status, and that dominant strategies for coping with threats to identity are maladaptive and focus largely on self-isolation and concealment of HIV status.

In Chapter 3, it was suggested that stressors, such as transphobia, sexism, and racism, can threaten identity, but that the relationship between these stressors and identity threat is likely to be mediated by the availability of social support. In other words, the more social support one can access, the less likely it is that one will experience threat and that identity threat will be acute. Much psychological research into coping with psychological adversity highlights the effectiveness of social support (Jaspal, 2018; Sani, Herrera, Wakefield, Boroch, & Gulyas, 2012). Yet, it was quite clear that the trans women who participated in this study had either limited or no access to social support. Many had attempted to share aspects of their identity with others over the life course but had encountered negative reactions, such as stigma and violence, and therefore refrained from disclosing their problems to others. The strategy of identity concealment and self-isolation was deemed to be preferable to the risk of violence and identity threat.

In this study, it has been shown that the self-esteem principle of identity is most susceptible to threat, given the multi-layered stigma faced by trans women and the internalisation of this stigma clearly evidenced in the data (Crocker & Major, 2003). Individuals may feel unable to derive a positive self-conception on the basis of identity, consisting of their transness, and HIV-positive status. Moreover, there were persistent threats to the continuity principle of identity (Breakwell, 1986), given that valued relationships either changed or were at risk when sensitive identity aspects (e.g. one's trans identity, HIV status) were disclosed to others. Although trans women living with HIV may conceal these identity aspects, they nevertheless fear their involuntary disclosure to others, which could introduce discontinuity in identity. The consistent accounts of stigma and rejection (on the basis of various identity elements) suggested that most interviewees also experienced a decreased sense of acceptance, inclusion and belonging—they simply felt that they did not 'fit in' (Mereish & Poteat, 2015). Moreover, as a result of perceived societal expectations, fear of stigma and the desire to 'fit in', trans women living with HIV may experience decreased identity authenticity (Vannini & Franzese, 2008). The data suggest that the experience of identity inauthenticity could threaten identity and challenge psychological wellbeing. It is plausible that both belonging and authenticity constitute additional identity principles which are potentially important to trans women (living with HIV) and susceptible to threat due to their lived experience.

Trans women living with HIV are struggling to construct an identity characterised by self-esteem, continuity, belonging and authenticity. Most interviewees reported previous self-identification as gay and had subsequently assimilated and accommodated their transness in their identity. While they evaluated their trans identity positively, some participants did not yet feel comfortable about manifesting this identity publicly because of anticipated stigma and, thus, potential threats to self-esteem (Turan et al., 2017). Chronic exposure to stigma across the life course led some to develop a sense of hypervigilance when interacting with others in that they anticipated stigma and sometimes misattributed innocuous events and situations to stigma. This could make social interactions and the formation of relationships difficult. Sex work was perceived to be widespread among trans women and all of the interviewees reported having engaged in sex work at some point during their lives. For some, sex work had become an important element of identity because of the financial benefits and 'escape' from poverty and dependence on others that it provided (Nadal, Davidoff, & Fujii-Doe, 2014). In some contexts, it enhanced self-efficacy while, in others, it had the potential to threaten authenticity since it entailed the requirement to engage in activities that were inconsistent with their identity.

There appears to be a struggle between maintaining a sense of authenticity and protecting self-esteem by deflecting stigma (which may result from authentic self-presentation as an HIV-positive trans woman). The balance between these two motivational principles is not consistently achieved. Moreover, their HIV status, an additional identity element, which was not generally assimilated and accommodated in identity, constituted a source of social stigma and threats to self-esteem, belonging and continuity. Most interviewees had not yet come to terms with their positive serostatus. Consistent with the Health Adversity Risk Model, it is clear that identity threat can induce negative affect (e.g. guilt, shame and anxiety), which itself can undermine psychological wellbeing outcomes. For some, this was so acute that it led to suicidal ideation or even suicide attempts. Unresolved identity threat, where few coping strategies are available, can lead to poor mental health and poor HIV outcomes (Jaspal, 2018).

A key finding in this study was that respondents felt uncomfortable about disclosing their HIV status to other people due to anticipated stigma. This in turn meant that they were unable to derive social support from others and that they remained at risk of decreased identity authenticity. In order to conceal their HIV status, individuals must 'pass' as HIV-negative, that is, to feign a negative serostatus on false pretences. Some decide not to disclose their HIV status to sexual partners, who in turn may insist on condomless sex with them. This can increase the risk of onward HIV transmission.

Furthermore, it is clear that some express trepidation about engaging with HIV services and about initiating and adhering to ART, because they are concerned about involuntary disclosure of their HIV status. This poses significant risks not only to their physical health but also their mental health. There is empirical evidence that trans people experience poorer mental health outcomes than the general population due partly to stigma and rejection (McNeil, Bailey, Ellis, Morton, & Regan, 2012). However, those living with HIV, many of whom have not disclosed their HIV status to others and do not access social support, are at especially high risk of poor mental health. Indeed, some respondents reported feeling lonely, distressed and even suicidal. The risk of poor mental health is significant not least due to the negative impact for engagement with HIV care, adherence to HIV treatment, and sexual health outcomes in trans women with poor mental health (Jaspal, 2018).

RECOMMENDATIONS AND FUTURE DIRECTIONS

There are several limitations to the EXTRA Study, which should be addressed in future research. First, the sample included only two visible ethnic minority individuals, although half of the participants were born outside the UK. It is known that trans people of ethnic minority background are especially affected by HIV and that they may face a unique set of challenges. This significant subgroup of trans women should be the focus of future research. Second, this study was intended to be an exploratory investigation of an under-researched, yet key population in the HIV epidemic, which has yielded rich qualitative insights into their identities and experiences. However, the findings are of course not generalisable to trans women living with HIV in the UK. Therefore, quantitative research with larger sample sizes should be conducted in the future in order to develop a more comprehensive profile of the identities and experiences of trans women. Third, in this volume, a social psychological approach was taken to shed light on trans women's experiences of living with HIV. While this approach attempts to marry individual and collective perspectives, it would be beneficial to conduct studies in this area from other disciplinary perspectives, such as sociology and anthropology. This would provide a more detailed and comprehensive account of HIV and trans women.

In any case, this preliminary qualitative study of trans women living with HIV in the UK does enable us to present a series of recommendations.

First, trans people should be much more visible in HIV prevention campaigns and HIV care initiatives, since several interviewees reported never feeling that they were at risk or that HIV was a concern and, after their diagnosis, did not consistently feel that services were inclusive of their identity.

Second, there is a need for a clear and coherent approach to stigma reduction. Interviewees unanimously reported facing multiple layers of stigma in relation to their transness, HIV status and involvement in sex work. Stigma is known to have insidious effects for identity, wellbeing and health. It also leads trans women to conceal their identity and to self-isolate, essentially depriving them of social support. Visibility performs an important function for stigma reduction. Robust equality and diversity training for healthcare professionals would be advantageous. Awareness-raising of trans identity in the general public would help demystify what remains a largely invisible and poorly understood group in society.

Third, as indicated in the Health Adversity Risk Model, both the availability of social support and the practitioner, in part, determine the choice of coping strategy that is adopted by people at risk. Healthcare practitioners have an important role to play in the health and wellbeing of trans people living with HIV. They should be mindful of the high prevalence of minority stressors (such as stigma, transphobic, structural violence, physical violence) among trans women, which may shape their level of risk, choice of coping strategy and level of engagement with HIV care. The clinical interventions that they offer should be cognisant of the relevant risk factors. Patients' experience of, and exposure to, these stressors should be probed sensitively. Although social support is one of the most effective and sustainable strategies for coping with psychological adversity, it is evident that not all trans women living with HIV can or wish to access it, for whatever reason. Some interviewees lamented the absence of an HIV support group specifically for trans women, while others did not wish to disclose their HIV status to other trans women and, thus, resisted this. HIV support groups should exist for those who wish to be involved in them. Trans women living with HIV should also be signposted to other potential sources of social support, which might reduce the reliance on identity concealment and self-isolation. The key objective should be to discourage identity concealment and self-isolation among trans women living with HIV.

Concluding Thoughts

In this volume, it has been shown that trans women living with HIV face multifaceted stigma, a complex relationship between sex work and their HIV status, and employ self-isolation and concealment of HIV status as prime strategies for coping with identity threat. In 2019, the British Association for Sexual Health and HIV Working Group produced a series of recommendations for integrated sexual health and HIV services for trans including non-binary people. It is hoped that the observations made in this volume will inform the development and implementation of these important clinical recommendations. Specifically, the social and psychological barriers to disclosing HIV status, accessing HIV care, and engaging with ART must be acknowledged. The risk of ineffective coping amid isolation and loneliness must be addressed. The complex identities of trans women living with HIV must be understood. In short, it is important that HIV care providers recognise the unique challenges that trans women living with HIV face, and the potential ways in which these challenges can inhibit access to HIV care and undermine health outcomes in this vulnerable population.

REFERENCES

Breakwell, G. M. (1986). *Coping with threatened identities*. London: Methuen.

British Association for Sexual Health and HIV. (2019). *BASHH recommendations for integrated sexual health services for trans, including non-binary people*. http://www.gpone.wales.nhs.uk/sitesplus/documents/1000/bashh-recommendations-for-integrated-sexual-health-services-for-trans-including-non-binary-people-2019pdf.pdf.

Crocker, J., & Major, B. (2003). The self-protective properties of stigma: Evolution of a modern classic. *Psychological Inquiry, 14*, 232–237. https://doi.org/10.1080/1047840X.2003.9682885.

Jaspal, R. (2018). *Enhancing sexual health, self-identity and wellbeing among men who have sex with men: A guide for practitioners*. London: Jessica Kingsley Publishers.

McNeil, J., Bailey, L., Ellis, S., Morton, J., & Regan, M. (2012). *Trans mental health and emotional wellbeing study 2012*. Scottish Transgender Alliance. http://www.scottishtrans.org/wp-content/uploads/2013/03/trans_mh_study.pdf.

Mereish, E., & Poteat, V. (2015). A relational model of sexual minority mental and physical health: The negative effects of shame on relationships, loneliness, and health. *Journal of Counseling Psychology, 62*(3), 425–437. https://doi.org/10.1037/cou0000088.

Nadal, K., Davidoff, K., & Fujii-Doe, W. (2014). Transgender women and the sex work industry: Roots in systemic, institutional, and interpersonal discrimination. *Journal of Trauma & Dissociation, 15*(2), 169–183. https://doi.org/10.1080/15299732.2014.867572.

Sani, F., Herrera, M., Wakefield, J. R. H., Boroch, O., & Gulyas, C. (2012). Comparing social contact and group identification as predictors of mental health. *British Journal of Social Psychology, 51*(4), 781–790. https://doi.org/10.1111/j.2044-8309.2012.02101.x.

Turan, B., Budhwani, H., Fazeli, P. L., Browning, W. R., Raper, J. L., Mugavero, M. J., & Turan, J. M. (2017). How does stigma affect people living with HIV? The mediating roles of internalized and anticipated HIV stigma in the effects of perceived community stigma on health and psychosocial outcomes. *AIDS and Behavior, 21*(1), 283–291. https://doi.org/10.1007/s10461-016-1451-5.

Vannini, P., & Franzese, A. (2008). The authenticity of self: Conceptualization, personal experience and practice. *Sociology Compass, 2*(5), 1621–1637. https://doi.org/10.1111/j.1751-9020.2008.00151.x.

INDEX